Global Neurosurgery

Editors

ROBERT J. DEMPSEY
MICHAEL M. HAGLUND

NEUROSURGERY
CLINICS OF NORTH AMERICA

www.neurosurgery.theclinics.com

Consulting Editors
RUSSELL R. LONSER
DANIEL K. RESNICK

October 2024 • Volume 35 • Number 4

ELSEVIER

1600 John F. Kennedy Boulevard • Suite 1800 • Philadelphia, Pennsylvania, 19103-2899

http://www.theclinics.com

NEUROSURGERY CLINICS OF NORTH AMERICA Volume 35, Number 4
October 2024 ISSN 1042-3680, ISBN-13: 978-0-443-12931-5

Editor: Stacy Eastman
Developmental Editor: Akshay Samson

Neurosurgery Clinics of North America (ISSN 1042-3680) is published quarterly by Elsevier Inc., 360 Park Avenue South, New York, NY 10010-1710. Months of issue are January, April, July, and October. Business and Editorial Offices: 1600 John F. Kennedy Blvd., Suite 1800, Philadelphia, PA 19103-2899. Customer Service Office: 11830 Westline Industrial Drive, St. Louis, MO 63146. Periodicals postage paid at New York, NY, and additional mailing offices. Subscription prices are $465.00 per year (US individuals), $499.00 per year (Canadian individuals), $579.00 per year (international individuals), $100.00 per year (US students), $255.00 per year (international students), and $100.00 per year (Canadian students). For institutional access pricing please contact Customer Service via the contact information below. International air speed delivery is included in all *Clinics* subscription prices. All prices are subject to change without notice. Orders, claims, and journal inquiries: Please visit our Support Hub page https://service.elsevier.com for assistance.

Reprints. For copies of 100 or more, of articles in this publication, please contact the Commercial Reprints Department, Elsevier Inc., 360 Park Avenue South, New York, NY 10010-1710. Tel. 212-633-3874; Fax: 212-633-3820; E-mail: reprints@elsevier.com.

Neurosurgery Clinics of North America is covered in *MEDLINE/PubMed (Index Medicus), EMBASE/Excerpta Medica, and Current Contents/Clinical Medicine (CC/CM).*

Contributors

CONSULTING EDITORS

RUSSELL R. LONSER, MD
Professor and Chair, Department of
Neurological Surgery, The Ohio State
University Wexner Medical Center, Columbus,
Ohio, USA

DANIEL K. RESNICK, MD, MS
Professor and Vice Chairman, Program
Director, Department of Neurosurgery,
University of Wisconsin-Madison School of
Medicine and Public Health, Madison,
Wisconsin, USA

EDITORS

ROBERT J. DEMPSEY, MD, FACS, FAANS
Professor, Chairman, Foundation for
International Education in Neurological Surgery
(FIENS); Manucher J. Javid Professor and
Chairman, Department of Neurological
Surgery, University of Wisconsin School of
Medicine and Public Health, Madison,
Wisconsin, USA

**MICHAEL M. HAGLUND, MD, PhD, MEd,
MACM, FAANS**
Distinguished Duke Professor of Neurosurgery,
Neurobiology, Global Health, and Orthopaedic
Surgery, Vice Chair of Education, Duke

Department of Neurosurgery, Division Chief,
Division of Global Neurosurery and Neurology,
Duke Global Neurosurgery and Neurology,
Duke University School of Medicine, Duke
University Global Health Institute, Duke
University, Department of Neurosurgery, Duke
Health, Professor, SingHealth Duke–NUS
Global Health Institute, Adjunct Professor
Barrow Global, Barrow Neurological Institute,
Program Director, Uganda Neurosurgery
Training Program, Durham, North Carolina,
USA

AUTHORS

ANASTASIA ARYNCHYNA-SMITH, MPH
Clinical Research Manager, Department of
Neurosurgery, Division of Pediatric
Neurosurgery, Children's of Alabama,
University of Alabama at Birmingham,
Birmingham, Alabama, USA

JAMES A. BALOGUN, MBBS
Consultant Neurological Surgeon, Division of
Neurosurgery, Department of Surgery, College
of Medicine, University of Ibadan, Ibadan,
Nigeria

MUSTAFA K. BASKAYA, MD
Professor, Department of Neurological
Surgery, University of Wisconsin School of
Medicine and Public Health, Madison,
Wisconsin, USA

JEFFREY BLOUNT, MD
Professor and Chief, Department of
Neurosurgery, Division of Pediatric
Neurosurgery, Children's of Alabama,
University of Alabama at Birmingham,
Birmingham, Alabama, USA

KATE BUNCH, MD
Resident, Department of Neurological Surgery,
University of Wisconsin School of Medicine
and Public Health, Madison, Wisconsin, USA

ROBERT J. DEMPSEY, MD, FACS, FAANS
Professor, Chairman, Foundation for
International Education in Neurological Surgery
(FIENS); Manucher J. Javid Professor and
Chairman, Department of Neurological
Surgery, University of Wisconsin School of

Medicine and Public Health, Madison, Wisconsin, USA

MICHAEL C. DEWAN, MD, MSCI
Assistant Professor, Department of Neurosurgery, Vanderbilt Institute for Global Health, Vanderbilt University Medical Center, Nashville, Tennessee, USA

YOSEF ELLENBOGEN, MD
Neurosurgery Resident, Division of Neurosurgery, Department of Surgery, University of Toronto, Toronto, Ontario, Canada

IGNATIUS N. ESENE, MD, PhD, MPH
Consultant Neurosurgeon, Foundation for International Education in Neurological Surgery (FIENS); Faculty of Health Sciences, University of Bamenda, Bambili, Cameroon; Winners Foundation, Yaounde, Cameroon

ANTHONY T. FULLER, MD, MScGH
External Advisor, Duke Global Neurosurgery and Neurology, Durham, North Carolina, USA; Fuller Health Solutions, Salt Lake City, Utah, USA

KEMEL A. GHOTME, MD, PhD
Associate Professor and Director, Translational Neuroscience Research Lab, Faculty of Medicine, Universidad de La Sabana, Chía, Colombia; Pediatric Neurosurgery, Department of Neurosurgery, Fundacion Santa Fe de Bogota, Bogota, Colombia

MARTINA GONZALEZ GOMEZ, MD, MSc
Global Neurosurgery Program Manager II, Department of Neurosurgery, Division of Pediatric Neurosurgery, Children's of Alabama, University of Alabama at Birmingham, Birmingham, Alabama, USA

GARRET P. GREENEWAY, MD
Neurosurgery Resident, Department of Neurological Surgery, University of Wisconsin School of Medicine and Public Health, Madison, Wisconsin, USA

SAKSHAM GUPTA, MD, MPH
Neurosurgery Resident and Global Surgery Fellow, Program for Global Surgery and Social Change, Department of Global Health and Social Medicine, Harvard Medical School, Department of Neurosurgery, Brigham and

Women's Hospital, Boston, Massachusetts, USA

MICHAEL M. HAGLUND, MD, PhD, MEd, MACM, FAANS
Distinguished Duke Professor of Neurosurgery, Neurobiology, Global Health, and Orthopaedic Surgery, Vice Chair of Education, Duke Department of Neurosurgery, Division Chief, Division of Global Neurosurery and Neurology, Duke Global Neurosurgery and Neurology, Duke University School of Medicine, Duke University Global Health Institute, Duke University, Department of Neurosurgery, Duke Health, Professor, SingHealth Duke–NUS Global Health Institute, Adjunct Professor Barrow Global, Barrow Neurological Institute, Program Director, Uganda Neurosurgery Training Program, Durham, North Carolina, USA

JOSELINE HAIZEL-COBBINA, MBChB, MPH
Population/Public Health Manager for Vanderbilt Global Neurosurgery Program, Department of Neurosurgery, Vanderbilt Institute for Global Health, Vanderbilt University Medical Center, Nashville, Tennessee, USA

RADZI HAMZAH, MD, MPH
Global Surgery Research Fellow, Program in Global Surgery and Social Change, Department of Global Health and Social Medicine, Harvard Medical School, Boston, Massachusetts, USA

JOSHUA R. HARPER, PhD
Professor of Engineering, Facultad de Ciencias de la Ingeniería, Universidad Paraguayo Alemana, Research Professor, Facultad de Informática, Universidad Comunera, Asunción, Paraguay

ROGER HARTL, MD
Professor of Neurological Surgery, Weill Cornell Medicine Department of Neurosurgery, Och Spine, New York Presbyterian Hospital, New York, New York, USA

MOJGAN HODAIE, MD
Professor of Surgery, Greg Wilkins-Barrick Chair in International Surgery, Division of Neurosurgery, Department of Surgery, University of Toronto, Division of Brain,

Imaging and Behaviour, Krembil Research Institute, University Health Network, Institute of Medical Science, Temerty Faculty of Medicine, University of Toronto, Toronto, Ontario, Canada

WALTER D. JOHNSON, MD, MPH, MBA
Professor, Department of Neurosurgery, Loma Linda University, Loma Linda, California, USA; Mercy Ships, Garden Valley, Texas, USA

JAMES M. JOHNSTON, MD
Associate Professor and Director of Pediatric Neurosurgery Fellowship Program, Department of Neurosurgery, Division of Pediatric Neurosurgery, Children's of Alabama, University of Alabama at Birmingham, Birmingham, Alabama, USA

ABDULLAH KELES, MD
Scientist I, Department of Neurological Surgery, University of Wisconsin School of Medicine and Public Health, Madison, Wisconsin, USA

JOYCE KOUEIK, MD, MS
Resident Physician, Department of Neurological Surgery, University of Wisconsin, Madison, Wisconsin, USA

LARS MEISNER, MD
Neurosurgery Resident, Department of Neurological Surgery, University of Wisconsin, Madison, Wisconsin, USA

RICHARD MOSER, MD
Professor, Department of Neurological Surgery, UMass Chan Medical School, Worcester, Massachusetts, USA

KEE B. PARK, MD, MPH
Lecturer Director of Policy and Advocacy, Global Neurosurgery Initiative, Program for Global Surgery and Social Change, Department of Global Health and Social Medicine, Harvard Medical School, Harvard University, Boston, Massachusetts, USA

MOODY QURESHI, MBChB, MMed (Surgery), FCS-ECSA, FRCSEd(SN)
Chairman of the Neurological Society, Department of Neurosurgery, Aga Khan University Hospital, Nairobi, Kenya

JARED REESE, MD
Neurosurgery Resident, Henry Ford Health Department of Neurosurgery, Detroit, Michigan, USA

FAITH C. ROBERTSON, MD, MSc, MBA
Neurosurgery Resident, Department of Neurosurgery, Massachusetts General Hospital, Harvard Business School, Boston, Massachusetts, USA

JACK ROCK, MD, FACS
Neurosurgeon, Henry Ford Health Department of Neurosurgery, Detroit, Michigan, USA

BRANDON G. ROCQUE, MD, MS
Professor, Division of Pediatric Neurosurgery, Department of Neurosurgery, Children's of Alabama, University of Alabama at Birmingham, Birmingham, Alabama, USA

GAIL ROSSEAU, MD
Clinical Professor, Department of Neurological Surgery, George Washington University School of Medicine and Health Sciences, Washington, DC, USA; Adjunct Professor, Barrow Global, Barrow Neurological Institute, Phoenix, Arizona, USA

STEVEN J. SCHIFF, MD, PhD
Harvey and Kate Cushing Professor of Neurosurgery, Vice Chair for Global Health, Department of Neurosurgery, Professor of Epidemiology, Department of Epidemiology of Microbial Diseases, Yale University, New Haven, Connecticut, USA

JULIET SEKABUNGA, MD
Physician, Foundation for International Education in Neurological Surgery (FIENS); Mulago National Referral Hospital, Kampala, Uganda

NATHAN A. SHLOBIN, MD, MBA
Neurosurgery Resident, Department of Neurosurgery, Neurological Institute of New York, New York Presbyterian Hospital, Columbia University Irving Medical Center, New York, New York, USA

SARAH WOODROW, MD
Staff Neurosurgeon and Director, Department of Neurological Surgery, Cleveland Clinic, Akron, Ohio, USA

JULIE WOODFIELD, PhD, FRCS, MSc, MBChB, BSc
Neurosurgeon, Centre for Clinical Brain Sciences, University of Edinburgh, Edinburgh, United Kingdom; Muhimbili Orthopaedic Institute, Dar es Salaam, Tanzania; Weill Cornell Medicine Department of Neurosurgery, New York, New York, USA

Contents

Preface: Service Through Education: Inspiring a Generation of Change in Global Neurosurgery   xiii

Robert J. Dempsey and Michael M. Haglund

An Overview of Global Neurosurgery   389

Joseline Haizel-Cobbina, James A. Balogun, Kee B. Park, Michael M. Haglund, Robert J. Dempsey, and Michael C. Dewan

Until recently, surgery had been passed over in the domain of global health, historically being described as "the neglected stepchild of global health." Knowledge of the existing global disparities in neurosurgical care has led to neurosurgery capacity-building efforts especially in low-income and middle-income countries. While many global collaborative projects are currently undertaken with philanthropic support, sustainability and scalability are not likely without governmental adoption of neurosurgery-inclusive national surgical plans. Momentum grows for the global neurosurgery community to develop a global neurosurgery action plan outlining goals, a guiding framework, an execution plan, and indicators for monitoring and evaluation.

The Role of Policy in Global Neurosurgery   401

Faith C. Robertson, Kee B. Park, and Walter D. Johnson

There have been tremendous strides over the past decade to institute strong policy as means to facilitate alignment on goals and strategies for global neurosurgical systems strengthening. In this chapter, we highlight key historic policy milestones in the global neurosurgery movement. We discuss the role of international organizations in neurosurgery, and the incorporation of neurosurgery into global health agendas. We then delve into specific examples of policies that have been established (such as comprehensive recommendations for neurotrauma, spina bifida, and hydrocephalus), highlight the role of international organizations in shaping neurosurgical policies, emphasize the importance of advocacy, and explore future directions.

Neurosurgical Advocacy in the Prevention of Neural Tube Defects: Impacting Global Fortification Policies Through Leadership, Collaboration, and Stakeholder Engagement   411

Nathan A. Shlobin, Kemel A. Ghotme, Anastasia Arynchyna-Smith, Martina Gonzalez Gomez, Sarah Woodrow, Jeffrey Blount, and Gail Rosseau

The G4 Alliance and its member organizations formed a delegation that participated in the 76th World Health Assembly (WHA) in 2023, which unanimously adopted the resolution to address micronutrient deficiencies through safe, effective food fortification to prevent congenital disorders such as spina bifida and anencephaly, the first neurosurgery-led resolution since the founding of the World Health Organization. The WHA included other resolutions and side events by the G4 Alliance and other organizations relevant to neurosurgery. An opportunity exists for neurosurgeons to harness the momentum from this resolution to promote initiatives to prevent neurosurgical disease or expand access to neurosurgical care.

Partnering in Global Health: What Is a Successful Dyad? The Duke Experience   421

Anthony T. Fuller and Michael M. Haglund

This article explores the transformative partnership between Duke Global Neurosurgery and Neurology (DGNN) and Uganda, emphasizing the power of dyads in international collaboration. It details the partnership's focus on service, research, and training, highlighting key accomplishments like the establishment of a neurosurgery residency program, expansion of services, and an epilepsy clinic. Challenges such as resource constraints and cross-cultural collaboration are addressed. Recommendations are provided for developing similar partnerships, underlining the importance of mutual respect, shared goals, and long-term commitment. The DGNN-Uganda dyad is a blueprint for leveraging collaboration to improve global neurosurgical care and reduce health care inequities.

Education and Training in Global Neurosurgery: Current State and Path Toward a Uniform Curriculum   429

Nathan A. Shlobin, Yosef Ellenbogen, Mojgan Hodaie, and Gail Rosseau

Education is a sustainable long-term measure to address the global burden of neurosurgical disease. Neurosurgery residencies in high-income countries are accredited by a regional governing body and incorporate various educational activities. Few opportunities for training may be present in low-income and middle-income countries due to a lack of neurosurgery residency programs, tuition, and health care workforce reductions. Core components of a neurosurgical training curriculum include operative room experience, clinical rounds, managing inpatients, and educational conferences. A gold standard for neurosurgical education is essential for creating comprehensive training experience, though training must be contextually appropriate.

Continuing Education for Global Neurosurgery Graduates: Visiting Surgeons, Skills Teaching, Bootcamps, and Twinning Programs   439

Julie Woodfield, Jared Reese, Roger Hartl, and Jack Rock

Neurosurgeons require post-graduate training to deliver safe, effective, and evidence-based care; to continually improve and adapt their methods through assessing the effect of their care and patient outcomes; and to train the future neurosurgeons of tomorrow to surpass current standards of care. We describe methods used by global collaborations to address these training needs on a worldwide scale, their risks, and their perceived benefits.

Establishing Microsurgery Skills Laboratories in Low- and Middle-income Countries with Integrated Remote Teaching: A Novel Approach   449

Abdullah Keles, Garret P. Greeneway, Robert J. Dempsey, and Mustafa K. Baskaya

Microneurosurgical techniques remain crucial for managing neurosurgical diseases, especially in low- and middle-income countries (LMICs) where other advanced treatment modalities are not available. The global distribution of these techniques is uneven due to disparities in infrastructure, equipment, and training. Medical professionals from LMICs face barriers in reaching training centers in high-income countries, as well as in accessing microsurgical techniques. To address these disparities in microsurgery training, we offer free and accessible microsurgery training model by combining the donations of microsurgery kits with a comprehensive support system that includes live-streamed, offline, and in-person assistance within LMICs.

Partnering with Foundations, Philanthropy, and Universities with Programs Supported by Local Physicians and Eventually Local Physicians Taking Ownership   465

Radzi Hamzah, Kate Bunch, Moody Qureshi, Kee B. Park, Michael M. Haglund, and Robert J. Dempsey

This article provides a thorough analysis of the evolution and current state of global neurosurgery, emphasizing the transformative power of partnerships between various stakeholders to address the stark inequities in neurosurgical care, especially in LMICs. It discusses the transition from reliance on short-term medical missions to the development of sustainable, locally led neurosurgical programs through education, training, and infrastructure development. The article highlights the importance of long-term educational exchanges, innovative digital learning platforms, and strategic collaborations with foundations, philanthropic organizations, and academic institutions to build local capacities, enhance global neurosurgical competency, and promote self-sufficiency in neurosurgical care across different regions.

Nongovernmental Organizations in Global Neurosurgery: Foundation for International Education in Neurological Surgery and Solidarity Bridge   475

Joyce Koueik, Lars Meisner, Brandon G. Rocque, Richard Moser, and Robert J. Dempsey

Health care disparities between high-income countries (HICs) and low- and middle-income countries (LMICs) are well established. The focus of the surgical aspect of health was identified in the early twenty-first century, and efforts to provide safe surgical intervention require the shift of resources from HICs to LMICs with specialized surgeons, anesthesiologists, and equipment. This intervention may make a difference on the short run; however, to achieve a long-term self-sustaining surgical service in the region of need, education and training of local physicians is key.

Engineering Principles and Bioengineering in Global Health   481

Joshua R. Harper and Steven J. Schiff

Medical technology plays a significant role in the reduction of disability and mortality due to the global burden of disease. The lack of diagnostic technology has been identified as the largest gap in the global health care pathway, and the cost of this technology is a driving factor for its lack of proliferation. Technology developed in high-income countries is often focused on producing high-quality, patient-specific data at a cost high-income markets can pay. While machine learning plays an important role in this process, great care must be taken to ensure appropriate translation to clinical practice.

Global Partnerships in Neurosurgery: Mapping the Need   489

Saksham Gupta, Martina Gonzalez Gomez, James M. Johnston, and Kee B. Park

The field of global neurosurgery seeks to improve access to neurosurgery and reduce health disparities worldwide. This process depends on intensive collaboration between partners in high-income and low-to-middle income country (LMIC) settings. Several such collaborations have propelled global neurosurgery forward, and long-standing partnerships in particular have brought subspecialty care and training to new locations. Recently, there have been more reports of collaborations between

LMICs themselves. In this narrative study, we summarize the state of collaboration in global neurosurgery and discuss how the field is likely to change moving forward.

Postgraduate Fellowships, Distant Continuing Education, and Funding in Neurosurgical Education   499

Ignatius N. Esene, Juliet Sekabunga, and Robert J. Dempsey

Neurosurgical education and training are the essential tenets for the development of a sustainable workforce. However, opportunities for training are limited in most parts of the world due to socioeconomic constraints and an inadequate workforce. This global deficit has triggered a huge drive to expand training opportunities. Although training programs are increasing numerically, most of these programs focus on basic residency training with no opportunities for fellowships and continuing education. Herein, we use the Foundation of International Education in Neurological Surgery as a global success model to elucidate on the role of fellowships, distant continuing education, and funding in neurosurgery.

Training the Next Generation of Academic Neurosurgeons in Global Health, Academics, and Research   509

Anthony T. Fuller and Michael M. Haglund

This article delves into academic global neurosurgeons' role in addressing the inequities in neurosurgical care globally. It outlines a comprehensive training framework incorporating global health education, research, and leadership development into neurosurgery residency programs. The article highlights the importance of interdisciplinary collaboration, cultural humility, and sustainable partnerships and advocates for a holistic approach to global neurosurgery. It underscores the necessity of integrating global health principles into neurosurgical training and practice, aiming to cultivate a new generation of neurosurgeons equipped to tackle the complex health challenges of our interconnected world.

NEUROSURGERY CLINICS OF NORTH AMERICA

FORTHCOMING ISSUES

January 2025
Controversies in Neurosurgery: 2025
Russell R. Lonser and Daniel K. Resnick, *Editors*

April 2025
Adult Hydrocephalus and Intracranial Pressure Disorders
Mark Hamilton, *Editor*

July 2025
Neurocritical Care of Trauma
P.B. Raksin and Laura B. Ngwenya, *Editors*

RECENT ISSUES

July 2024
Disorders and Treatment of the Cerebral Venous System
Shahid M. Nimjee, *Editor*

April 2024
New Technologies in Spine Surgery
Adam S. Kanter and Nicholas Theodore, *Editors*

January 2024
Epilepsy Surgery: Paradigm Shifts
Jimmy C. Yang and R. Mark Richardson, *Editors*

SERIES OF RELATED INTEREST

Neurologic Clinics
https://www.neurologic.theclinics.com/
Neuroimaging Clinics
https://www.neuroimaging.theclinics.com/

THE CLINICS ARE AVAILABLE ONLINE!
Access your subscription at:
www.theclinics.com

Preface

Service Through Education: Inspiring a Generation of Change in Global Neurosurgery

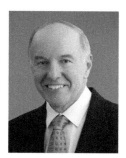
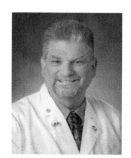

Robert J. Dempsey, MD, FACS, FAANS Michael M. Haglund, MD, PhD, MEd, MACM, FAANS

Editors

Global neurosurgery will define the relevance and future of the entire field of neurosurgery. Neurosurgery as it stands now is a very small component, as low as 1% of the field of medicine. To be relevant, it needs to go where the patients are, and that means addressing the imperative issue of providing care to the vast majority of the world, believed to be as many as 5.5 billion people, who do not now have access to specialized neurosurgical care and need it. In this issue, Global Neurosurgery, we examine the extent of this problem and the repercussions for society of having the majority of people not have access to lifesaving neurosurgical procedures. Without such access, there can be no complete/effective trauma system, no adequate cancer or stroke care, no adequate treatment of pain or congenital anomalies of children. The implications are quite clear. Solutions to this problem will not come from expecting the present small number of neurosurgeons to travel throughout the regions to provide the care, nor will it come from draining the brightest people from the regions of need and training them elsewhere without supplying the infrastructure that will allow them to succeed in their native lands. In these articles of *Neurosurgery Clinics of North America*, the authors address education as

the basis of a solution to correct this disparity. In this issue, education and training are looked at, including the important roles of policy and advocacy in prevention and of how, through partnering with established programs and neurosurgical societies, self-sustaining training programs can be developed both regionally and in individual countries and areas of need. These articles also highlight modern technology, such as establishing microsurgical skills laboratories in the countries of need and bringing established educational aids, such as boot camps, twinning programs, and visiting professors, to help to support the needs. The issue also continues to show how we will be able to track this with modern technology and how this technology can not only provide continuing education but also actually bring us into the operating rooms in real time to assure training continues throughout the career and enhances the possibility that the people trained will be trainers themselves, taking care of patients long into the future.

In this issue, readers will find some of the brightest minds in this field bringing their expertise and unique facets of service in education to the problem. The major takeaways are that despite what appears to be a daunting worldwide need for

Neurosurg Clin N Am 35 (2024) xiii–xiv
https://doi.org/10.1016/j.nec.2024.07.001
1042-3680/24/© 2024 Published by Elsevier Inc.

specialized neurosurgical care, solutions are possible through the energy of outstanding and humanitarian leadership, which is dedicated not to impose systems but rather to develop within the area of need the champions and expertise that will lead these programs. A true self-sustaining program should be of and by the people they serve. This allows the governmental and societal support that is needed for successful partnering to a solution. Examples of success, such as in prevention of neural tube deficits, show the strength of collaboration—be it with the government, with neurosurgical colleagues, or with a society or population that we serve. In the end, neurosurgery has identified a great and global need but should not be daunted, as through collaboration solutions are possible and imperative.

It is our hope that the issue will not only provide a roadmap for change and improvement in care but also inspire that just as solutions must require collaboration from many, the ability to participate is present in all of us. Each in our own way brings a strength to problems. That strength can be infectious and, ultimately, successful. We hope that you find this issue both educational and inspiring, offering possible solutions to what once seemed to be an impossible task, but now we truly believe is not only necessary, but possible.

Thank you.

Robert J. Dempsey, MD, FACS, FAANS
Department of Neurological Surgery
University of Wisconsin School of Medicine and
Public Health
600 Highland Avenue
Madison, WI 53792, USA

Michael M. Haglund, MD, PhD, MEd, MACM,
FAANS
Duke Department of Neurosurgery
Duke Global Neurosurgery and Neurology
SingHealth Duke–NUS Global Health Institute
Barrow Neurological Institute
Uganda Neurosurgery Training Program
Durham, NC, USA

E-mail addresses:
dempsey@neurosurgery.wisc.edu (R.J. Dempsey)
michael.haglund@duke.edu (M.M. Haglund)

An Overview of Global Neurosurgery

Check for updates

Joseline Haizel-Cobbina, MBChB, MPH[a,b], James A. Balogun, MBBS[c], Kee B. Park, MD, MPH[d], Michael M. Haglund, MD, PhD, MEd, MACM[e], Robert J. Dempsey, MD[f], Michael C. Dewan, MD, MSCI[a,b,*]

KEYWORDS

- Global neurosurgery • Health disparities • Neurosurgical care • Education and training • Research
- Collaborations

KEY POINTS

- About 23 million people worldwide are estimated to suffer from neurosurgical conditions annually with close to 14 million requiring surgical intervention.
- Global neurosurgical inequity is not only limited to low-income and middle-income countries (LMICs) or the Global South, but also exists in high-income countries (HICs).
- A multifaceted approach has been adopted to address the existing disparities in neurosurgical care largely driven by collaborative efforts between HIC and LMIC neurosurgeons and institutions.
- Adopting a systems-based approach with the engagement of all stakeholders including public officials, administrators, surgeons, and patients will help ensure sustainable, patient-centered success in global neurosurgery.

BACKGROUND

Until recently, surgery had been passed over in the domain of global health, historically being described as "the neglected stepchild of global health."[1] The launch of the Lancet Commission on Global Surgery in January 2014 brought about a paradigm shift in global health practice incorporating surgical and anesthetic care.[2] The surge in health conditions requiring surgical intervention globally, with a greater burden in low-income and middle-income countries (LMICs), warrants urgent attention as the global health community strives to achieve the Sustainable Development Goals for 2030.[3] At the inaugural meeting of the Lancet Commission on Global Surgery, Dr Jim Yong Kim, the 12th President of the World Bank, called for the address of inequity in global surgical care, stating that "surgery is an indivisible, indispensable part of health care."[4] The resolution passed by the World Health Assembly (WHA) in 2015 on "Strengthening Emergency and Essential Surgical Care and Anesthesia as a Component of Universal Health Coverage" corroborates this call to action.[5] The enhanced focus on the delivery of safe, effective, and affordable surgical care cuts across multiple surgical subspecialties including neurosurgery.[6,7]

Roughly 23 million people worldwide are estimated to suffer from neurosurgical conditions annually with close to 14 million requiring surgical intervention, forming a significant proportion of the overall global surgical disease burden.[2,8] Building on the proposed definition for global surgery by

[a] Department of Neurosurgery, Vanderbilt University Medical Center, Nashville, TN, USA; [b] Vanderbilt Institute for Global Health, Vanderbilt University Medical Center, Nashville, TN, USA; [c] Division of Neurosurgery, Department of Surgery, College of Medicine, University of Ibadan, Ibadan, Nigeria; [d] Program in Global Surgery and Social Change, Harvard University, Boston, MA, USA; [e] Department of Neurosurgery, Division of Global Neurosurgery and Neurology, Duke University School of Medicine, Durham, NC, USA; [f] Department of Neurological Surgery, School of Medicine and Public Health, University of Wisconsin, Madison, WI, USA
* Corresponding author. Division of Pediatric Neurological Surgery, Department of Neurological Surgery, Vanderbilt Children's Hospital, 2200 Children's Way, 9226 Doctors Office Tower, Nashville TN 37232-9557.
E-mail address: michael.dewan@vumc.org

Neurosurg Clin N Am 35 (2024) 389–400
https://doi.org/10.1016/j.nec.2024.05.001
1042-3680/24/© 2024 Elsevier Inc. All rights are reserved, including those for text and data mining, AI training, and similar technologies.

Dare and colleagues,[6] global neurosurgery has been defined as "an area for study, research, practice, and advocacy that places priority on improving health outcomes and achieving health equity for all people worldwide who are affected by neurosurgical conditions or have a need for neurosurgical care, with a special emphasis on underserved populations and populations in crisis."[9] Knowledge of the existing global disparities in neurosurgical care has led to focusing a majority of global neurosurgery capacity-building efforts in LMICs, wherein resides the greatest burden and need. However, it is worth noting that global neurosurgical inequity is not only limited to LMICs or the Global South, but also exists in high-income countries (HICs) with individuals with low socioeconomic status, racial/ethnic minorities, the uninsured, and those living in remote areas experiencing challenges with access to timely and adequate neurosurgical care.[6,10–13]

Global Burden of Neurosurgical Diseases

Essential neurosurgical conditions have been defined as "conditions in which treatment neglect would directly result in severe disability or death."[8] These include traumatic brain injury and traumatic spine injury, central nervous system (CNS) tumors, hydrocephalus, neural tube defects (NTDs), CNS infections, epilepsy, and cerebrovascular diseases.[8,14] LMICs bear about 80% of the essential disease burden with the remaining 20% arising in HICs.[8,14] Wide disparities also exist across World Health Organization (WHO) regions; roughly 40% of neurosurgical conditions are found in the South-East Asian Region and Africa Region.[8] Neurotrauma and cerebrovascular diseases are the major contributors to the global neurosurgical disease burden and are 2 of the leading causes of death according to a WHO report.[15] Neurotrauma is the leading cause of trauma-related injuries and trauma-related deaths worldwide with about 89% of such trauma burden deriving from LMICs.[15–17] Similarly, a higher prevalence of epilepsy is reported in LMICs compared to HICs, with an estimated 80% of people living with epilepsy located in LMICs.[18] Neurosurgical-oncologic care presents another area with stark disparities in both incidence of cases and treatment outcomes reported in HICs and LMICs. While a relatively higher incidence of CNS tumor cases are reported in HICs compared to LMICs, likely due to under diagnosis and underreporting in LMICs, higher mortality rates are reported in LMICs for both adult and pediatric populations.[19,20] The pediatric population is not exempted from the existing global disparities. Hydrocephalus and NTDs make up a significant proportion of the neurosurgical disease burden (7.3%) and are part of the leading causes of childhood morbidity and mortality.[20] Each year, 400,000 children are diagnosed with hydrocephalus out of which 75% are in LMICs.[21] Similarly, about 300,000 children are born with NTDs yearly with a higher birth prevalence in Africa (78/100,000) and Asia (81/100,000) compared to North America (37/100,000).[22]

Disparities in Neurosurgical Care

Neurosurgical care is expensive. Optimal treatment outcomes involve a collaborative effort among a multidisciplinary specialist teams which may include neurosurgeons, anesthesiologists, neurointensivists, neurologists, operating room personnel, pathologists, radiologists, emergency staff, nurses, and other ancillary health care providers. Beyond human resources, surgical infrastructure is costly and includes imaging technologies, surgical equipment, operating theaters, and recovery and intensive care facilities, among many others. Today, the distribution of human resource and surgical infrastructure across continents, countries, and regions is inequitable. Currently, there are roughly 50,000 neurosurgeons globally.[8,23,24] The existing neurosurgical workforce is inadequate to meet the demand of essential neurosurgical care worldwide, and this workforce deficit is expectedly most profound in LMICs. Indeed, more than 30 countries are without a single neurosurgeon.[8,24] Averaged across WHO regions, there were as few as 1 neurosurgeon per 2 million people in the African region, relative to 1 neurosurgeon per 82,700 people in the Western Pacific Region.[24] **Fig. 1** shows the disparities in the volume of essential neurosurgical conditions requiring surgical intervention based on the existing neurosurgical workforce across different WHO regions. In addition to the workforce shortage, LMICs have very limited surgical infrastructure which further hinders care.[23,25–27] Neurosurgical care also tends to be concentrated in urban areas with rural populations lacking timely access to care. Many patients thus have to travel long distances to seek neurosurgical care.[28] About a third of HIC patients need to travel more than 2 hours to seek emergency neurosurgical care; in LMICs that figure is closer to three-quarters.[28]

HISTORICAL STRATEGIES TO ADDRESS GLOBAL DISPARITIES IN NEUROSURGICAL CARE

A multifaceted approach has been developed over the last 6 decades to address the existing disparities in neurosurgical care largely driven by collaborative efforts between HIC and LMIC

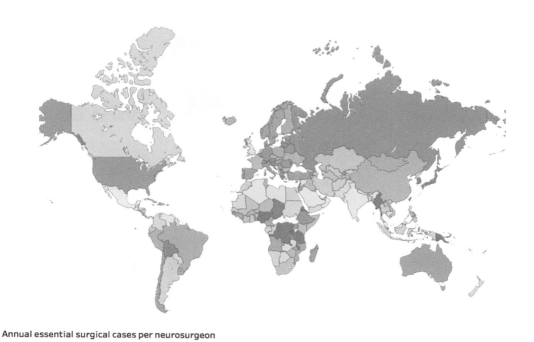

Annual essential surgical cases per neurosurgeon

0 ≥ 10,000

500

Fig. 1. A map showing the disparities in the volume of essential neurosurgical conditions requiring surgical intervention based on the existing neurosurgical workforce across different countries and World Health Organization regions. (*From* Dewan MC, Rattani A, Fieggen G, et al. Global neurosurgery: the current capacity and deficit in the provision of essential neurosurgical care. Executive Summary of the Global Neurosurgery Initiative at the Program in Global Surgery and Social Change. Journal of neurosurgery. 2018 Apr 2018;[8] with permission. © OpenStreetMap contributors.)

neurosurgeons and institutions.[29] Recently, collaborations have taken the format of partnerships and twinning programs established between HIC institutions and LMIC institutions.[30,31] These collaborations have largely involved HIC institutions in North America and Europe and LMIC institutions in Africa, South America and Southeast Asia with North American institutions leading a majority of the collaborative efforts.[7] Partnerships and twinning programs may vary in the scope of activities. **Fig. 2** outlines the range of collaborative activities in global neurosurgery partnerships targeted at capacity building in LMICs.

Humanitarian Initiatives Toward Provision of Neurosurgical Care

Neurosurgical missions and donation of equipment

Neurosurgical missions have possibly served as the oldest collaborative model with HIC neurosurgeons conducting short-term visits often with a multidisciplinary team to an LMIC site primarily to help address the surgical needs of the population.

Some mission trips have gradually evolved to include an education and training component for both neurosurgeons and ancillary health staff.[32] For many HIC neurosurgeons, mission trips have served as the firsthand exposure to the global inequities that exist in neurosurgical care and a catalyst for future involvement. While typically well-intentioned, short-term missions have received criticism for incongruent visitor-host goals, patchy or absent clinical follow-up, and methodologies that lack sustainability. Nonetheless, neurosurgical missions have also provided an avenue for the donation of surgical equipment and supplies. Outside of clinical missions, some organizations have undertaken medical equipment donation projects which involve collecting equipment and supplies from hospitals, medical device companies, and other donor institutions and distributing them to lower-resourced facilities. Millions of dollars' worth of equipment and medical supplies have been donated over the years.[33,34] Donations of equipment have been found to greatly improve the quality and safety of neurosurgical procedures in LMICs.[35,36]

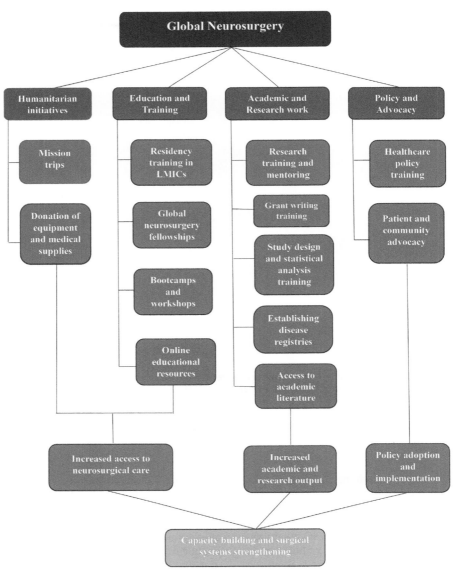

Fig. 2. A conceptual diagram showing the 4 domains and activities involved in global neurosurgery practice.

Low-cost devices and procedures
Medical devices—particularly implants—illustrate well the inequity that currently exists in neurosurgery worldwide. From inherently limited settings, there have been derived several examples of cost-effective solutions to common neurosurgical problems. As an example, the prohibitive cost of Western shunts driven by industry, tariffs, and high exchange rates challenged some LMIC neurosurgeons to devise locally made shunts for hydrocephalus treatment leading to the invention of the "Chhabra shunt" which received a patent in India in 1985 and the "Malawi shunt" in 1992.[37,38] The spectrum of the 'Chhabra shunt' has also been

progressively widened. Without access to rigid endoscopes, Dr Benjamin Warf pioneered an alternative treatment for hydrocephalus combining endoscopic third ventriculostomy (ETV) and choroid plexus cauterization (CPC) procedure using a flexible scope not typically meant for neurosurgery.[39,40] In a striking example of reverse innovation, the ETV/CPC procedure has become the standard of care for many patients with hydrocephalus worldwide. Beyond hydrocephalus treatment, LMIC neurosurgeons find creative ways to treat patients with other conditions using the limited resources available to them, many of which have not yet been documented.[39,41] A neurosurgeon in

South Africa has demonstrated the feasibility of using flexible endoscope to perform a flexible endoscope–assisted suture release for the management of sagittal synostosis in the absence of a rigid endoscope.[42]

Task Shifting and Task Sharing

Tasking shifting and task sharing (TS/S) in neurosurgery involves the act of delegating clinical tasks to non-neurosurgical specialists or nonphysician clinicians.[43] In task sharing, health care providers share clinical responsibilities and work together collaboratively to provide care to patients. On the other hand, task shifting is the delegation of the provision of neurosurgical care to non-neurosurgical specialists or nonphysician clinicians.[43] A recent global study exploring TS/S practices in neurosurgery showed that task sharing was largely preferred by both HIC and LMIC neurosurgeons to task shifting due to concerns of undue autonomy and poor clinical outcomes in the latter.[43] Additionally, LMIC neurosurgeons find task shifting to be professionally disruptive and can potentially cripple efforts to enhance neurosurgery training opportunities and access to safe and quality neurosurgical care.[44,45] Though TS/S is practiced in many LMICs out of necessity or desperation, it remains controversial, and calls have been made to standardize its implementation by defining the scope of clinical practice, standardizing training for providers involved, instituting competency-based evaluations, and maintenance of certification.[43]

Education and Training

Multidirectional education and training represent core components of global neurosurgery capacity building. A collaborative approach to neurosurgical training leads to the development of a well-structured curriculum best suited to meet the goals of the training program and enhance proficiency of trainees in different settings.[46,47] Many LMICs lack clinical neurosurgery training opportunities despite the need to increase the neurosurgery workforce; others lack subspecialty training opportunities within neurosurgery.[48] To address this challenge, the global neurosurgery community with the support of academic institutions, organizational societies, foundations, and donors has implemented many diverse training programs in both HICs and LMICs. Many of these will be discussed throughout this special issue.

Training opportunities in high-income countries

HIC-based training programs have been designed for LMIC neurosurgeons or residents to visit an academic institution for a finite time period to participate in clinical and/or research fellowship programs after which trainees return to their home countries to practice. Examples of HIC-based training programs include the Global Neurotrauma Fellowship by Barrow Neurological institute, Phoenix, AZ 85013, USA.[49] The University of Toronto, Canada, also offers a 12-month fellowship in neuro-oncology and skull base surgery and pediatric neurosurgery at the Toronto Western Hospital and The Hospital for Sick Children, respectively.[50] Many others exist. Through such programs, international fellows have the opportunity to share their experiences with faculty, residents, and co-fellows from around the world which further enriches the program. They spark lifelong connections and establish collaborations to aid capacity building in their home countries, meanwhile fostering leadership in organized neurosurgical societies. While there is no foolproof solution to the delicate issue of retention of exposed individuals/fellows in their home countries, efforts must continually be directed at reducing the factors that enkindle brain drain. Recruiting passionate individuals with a tendency to return and practice at home, intentionally directing the educational needs of the individuals to the uniqueness of their practice environment, and empowering LMIC surgeons with basic tools and equipment for clinical practice and research to mitigate some of the frustrations faced upon returning home.

Training opportunities in low-income and middle- income countries

Despite the benefits derived from training programs in HICs, access to neurosurgical training opportunities in LMICs remains paramount to addressing the workforce deficit in LMICs. National and regional-based trainings pioneered and led by local neurosurgeons in LMICs have provided veritable foundation for training neurosurgeons to meet local needs over the past decades.[51] A number of organizations and academic institutions have also played active roles in establishing and complementing training programs in LMICs. The World Federation of Neurosurgical Societies (WFNS) has instituted a sponsored postgraduate fellowship training program currently involving 27 centers in 15 countries for LMIC neurosurgeon graduates.[52] Two full residency training programs, WFNS-Rabat Training Center (Morocco) for training African neurosurgeons and the Recife WFNS Reference Training Center (Brazil) for training Portuguese-speaking and Spanish-speaking neurosurgeons, were established in 2002 and 2007, respectively, to help advance training efforts in low-resource settings.[52] Under the leadership of Professor Majid Samii, Project Africa100 was launched in 2014 to train 100 neurosurgeons in Africa to help meet the demands of the growing population. In line with this project, the WFNS also supports 6 additional regional training centers in Sub-Saharan Africa, South America, and Asia with neurosurgeon candidates drawn from various African countries.[53] The Foundation for International Education in Neurological Surgery (FIENS) has been actively engaged in training neurosurgeons around the world for more than 50 years.[9] FIENS currently has education and training programs in 27 country sites including the Tanzania Training Program, Duke East Africa Neurosurgery training Program, and Cambodia Neurosurgery Support Project.[9] The Duke East Africa Neurosurgery Training Program has trained 9 Ugandans with 20 more trainees in the program. These training programs have been developed in conjunction with academic institutions, foundations such as Meditech Foundation and Neurosurgery Education and Development Foundation, and local training boards such as the College of Surgeons of Central, East, and Southern Africa and the West African College of Surgeons.[46] FIENS also provides funding support for LMIC trainees to complete their training at a local or regional training center or to obtain specialized training at an HIC training center through the Clack and Bassett Fellowship programs.[54]

Bidirectional training
The success of capacity building efforts is heavily dependent on the degree of engagement and the compatibility between HIC-LMIC stakeholders.[55] Over the last couple decades, there has been an increasing number of neurosurgeons, trainees, and students with a desire to be actively involved in ongoing capacity-building efforts in LMICs. Now more than ever, it has become important to incorporate public health within a standard curriculum.[55,56] Beyond public health training, the shift toward a twinning paradigm with long-term partnerships between HIC and LMIC institutions offers the unique opportunity for a bidirectional global neurosurgery training paving the way for Global North-to-Global South neurosurgeons and trainee interactions. A few academic institutions in the United States offer 9-month to 12-month global neurosurgery fellowship programs in East Africa including Duke University, Weill Cornell Medicine, and Barrow Neurologic Institute.[46] Many other institutions around the world also offer the opportunity to both LMIC and HIC trainees and medical students to join faculty on short-term trips or travel

independently to partner sites through their global neurosurgery programs. This offers neurosurgeons, trainees, and medical students the opportunity to learn from their cross-world colleagues, experience neurosurgical practice in different settings, and conduct research while also sharing their clinical and research knowledge and skillset with the local team. Such LMIC-HIC team interactions help foster cultural competency and effective community engagement.

Neurosurgical boot camps and training workshops
Neurosurgery residency and fellowship training programs are further enriched by a plenitude of training workshops, boot camps, and scientific sessions to enhance the clinical knowledge and management skills of neurosurgeons and trainees. The Society of Neurological Surgeons developed the international boot camp learning model and curriculum in 2010 in the United States.[57] This includes didactics, case discussions, skill stations, and simulations. The WFNS and FIENS has with various stakeholders including neurosurgical professional societies such as the European Association of Neurosurgical Societies (EANS), Congress of Neurological Surgeons, Asian Australasian Society of Neurosurgery, Asian Congress of Neurologic Surgeons, the Neurological Society of India, and the Sociedade Brasileira de Neurocirurgia to organize international training workshops and boot camps since 2015.[57,58] This is targeted at improving the management of multiple neurosurgical conditions including neurotrauma, tumors, epilepsy, congenital deformities, cerebrovascular conditions, infections, and acquired degenerative conditions.[58]

For more than a decade, CURE International, in collaboration with the International Federation for Spina Bifida and Hydrocephalus, implemented a neuroendoscopy training program in Uganda which trained and equipped dozens of LMIC neurosurgeons to better treat hydrocephalus.[59] The University of Alabama, Birmingham, USA established collaborations with Vietnam aimed at expanding pediatric neurosurgery capacity. The training model developed involves in-country hands-on training, fellowship training at the HIC partner site, and continuous mentorship using virtual presence technology.[60] The coronavirus disease 2019 pandemic saw the launch of NeuroKids Inc which implemented the advanced training program in pediatric neurosurgery using virtual presence technology to improve hydrocephalus care in LMICs. This hybrid training model includes a short-term on-site training on neuroendoscopic management of hydrocephalus followed by remote surgical training over a 12-month period using virtual presence technology (**Fig. 3**A, B).

Online Educational Resources

The use of electronic media to facilitate teaching and learning (e-learning) has been adopted at every level of education including medical and surgical training.[61] Within neurosurgery, the advent of the digital era and the increasing Internet penetration in LMICs have created an unprecedented opportunity to foster global collaborations and enhance training.[62] While countless online resources exist, some of the most popular ones include the Neurosurgical Atlas,[63] the Rhoton Collection (available on the American Association of Neurologic Surgeons Neurosurgery YouTube channel),[64] 3D Neuroanatomy,[65] UpSurgeOn,[66] Brainbook,[67] Touch Surgery,[68] and the International Society for Pediatric Neurosurgery (ISPN) Guide to Pediatric Neurosurgery.[69] Other online resources include the Neurosurgery Education and Training School created by the All India Institute of Medical Sciences which provides free educational materials, the Ptolemy Project which provides LMIC surgeons free access to journal articles, and the WFNS Young Neurosurgeons Forum Stream which shares educational content and provides networking opportunities.[9] Language and financial barriers are not immune to online educational materials, and the nature in which those barriers are navigated is likely to influence their reach and impact.

Web-Based Collaborations

Web-based collaborations form an essential medium through which collaborative work in global neurosurgery can flourish. InterSurgeon, a free virtual platform was created in 2017 with the support of ISPN to reduce barriers to information access and also develop and facilitate collaborative partnerships in global neurosurgery.[70,71] InterSurgeon currently partners with the G4 Alliance and has grown significantly with an expansion of its modules to cover other surgical and anesthesia specialties.[71] Mentors and trainees are matched on the online platform to facilitate education and training, clinical guidance for operative technique, and research activities.[72] NeuroMind is a mobile device application created to facilitate collaborations among neurosurgeons, neurologists, residents, and medical students interested in neuroscience.[73] NeuroMind, supported by the EANS, provides an interactive decision support for neurotrauma, neuro-oncology, and neurovascular case management.[73] VirtualBoard (Genomet, New York, USA) is a cloud-based platform which is used by a collaborative team of US-based and Kenya-based neurosurgeons for virtual tumor board meetings to discuss challenging neuro-oncology cases at Tenwek Hospital in Kenya.[74,75] "Virtual Visiting Professors" is an online education program series organized by FIENS for neurosurgery residents and recent graduates to augment traditional visiting professor lectures.[76]

Academic and research collaborations

The development and implementation of evidenced-based policies and clinical practice guidelines is largely dependent on quality research involving the target population. There is, however, a dearth of primary research from LMICs on neurotrauma, neuro-oncology, epilepsy, and hydrocephalus, among other entities.[21,25,77–82] There are also substantial disparities between HIC-led and LMIC-led neurosurgical clinical trials, with HICs leading majority of clinical trials.[83] Efforts to develop research capacity in LMICs through global neurosurgery collaborations are ongoing, and while major disparities remain, academic and research initiatives led by LMIC authors are growing.[7,78,84] Some of these research initiatives include the Global Neurosurgery Initiative of the Harvard Program in Global Surgery and Social Change

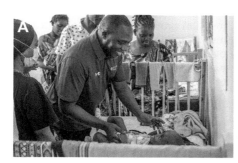
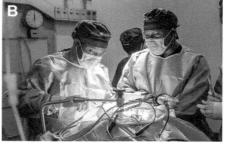

Fig. 3. (*A*) On daily ward rounds in Mombasa, Kenya, Dr Peter Ssenyonga (Neurosurgeon–Uganda) evaluates a postoperative patient. (*B*) A Kenyan neurosurgeon (*left*) receiving surgical training from an Ugandan colleague (*right*), in Mombasa, Kenya.

(PGSSC) which provides fellowship opportunities to LMIC residents with a focus on research, advocacy, and policy.[85] The National Institutes of Health Fogarty Global Health Training Program offers 12-month funded research fellowships in LMICs which is open to both US and LMIC postdoctoral fellows.[86] The National Institute for Health Research Global Health Research Group on Neurotrauma was established with the aim of increasing clinical research participation and improving neurotrauma outcomes in LMICs.[87] The Society for Neuro-Oncology Sub-Saharan Africa organizes monthly interactive webinars addressing neuro-oncology specialties, supportive care, and advocacy, all featuring speakers and participants from across the globe.[88] The Association of Future African Neurosurgeons has implemented a global neurosurgery research incubator program for aspiring academic global neurosurgeons in Africa which provides members at all career levels with mentorship, skills, and experience in research from study design to post-publication communication.[89] Many other collaborations exist and such opportunities are likely to grow as the neurosurgical global community grows closer.

Policy and Advocacy Initiatives

As the global surgery movement evolves, the global neurosurgery community continues to be actively engaged in policy and advocacy work aimed at scaling up surgical, obstetric, and anesthesia services globally as part of achieving equitable surgical care everywhere. The WFNS plays a crucial role in advocating for universal access to neurosurgical care and providing technical and strategic input for the WHO. Neurosurgeons play a fundamental role in international advocacy resulting in the WHA resolution focused on emergency and trauma care.[90] The Global Alliance for Prevention of Spina Bifida-F, a coalition of individuals and organizations co-founded by the G4 Alliance is actively working to introduce the WHA resolution for universal mandatory folic acid fortification of staple foods to promote global prevention of folic acid–preventable spina bifida and anencephaly.[91] The PGSSC in collaboration with the United Nations Institute for Training and Research and the Global Surgery Foundation is working with several ministries of health to develop and implement a national surgical, obstetric, and anesthesia plan that integrates plans to improve surgical access into their overall national health plan.[92] National neurosurgical societies—both in HIC and LMICs—are evolving to more intentionally incorporate the advocacy and engagement of government and the private sector

into their mandates; national societal meetings and national medical body representation are important vehicles to promote neurosurgical practice and training.[93] And each day in the clinics or in theater, whether in London or Lilongwe, neurosurgeons advocate for better health by delivering care to their patients.

BARRIERS TO THE GLOBAL NEUROSURGERY MOVEMENT

The barriers that exist for global neurosurgeons are the same as what stands in the way of the equitable delivery of safe and affordable health care worldwide. The expense of neurosurgical care and the perception of neurosurgery as a subspecialty commodity certainly add additional challenges. While many global collaborative projects are currently undertaken with philanthropic support, sustainability and scalability are not likely without governmental adoption of neurosurgery-inclusive national surgical plans. The scarcity of private funding for global surgery capacity-building projects limits the number and scope of projects. Public safety legislation and enforcement have been shown to mitigate neurosurgical trauma burden in many countries and settings.[94] Brain drain is a phenomenon which can further deplete an already limited neurosurgical workforce in LMICs.[50] The economic and political instability in some countries plays a role in the brain drain phenomenon. In relation to Global North-South collaborations, opportunity costs, loss of income, time constraints, inability to travel, language or cultural barriers, and personal safety have all been cited as barriers to active participation both among HIC and LMIC actors.[95]

FUTURE DIRECTIONS

With an alarming unmet burden of neurosurgical disease worldwide, the work ahead is as challenging as it is imperative. Teamwork, empathy, determination, and grace will be required. Momentum grows for the global neurosurgery community to develop a global neurosurgery action plan outlining goals, a guiding framework, an execution plan, and process and outcome indicators for monitoring and evaluation. Evaluation reports are to serve as a basis to reassess and improve on operations, outcomes, and systems processes in relation to the set goals of established partnerships. Adopting a systems-based approach with the engagement of all stakeholders including public officials, administrators, surgeons, and patients will help ensure sustainable, patient-centered success. An enormous amount of work lies ahead for our community as we work together to build neurosurgery capacity around the world, improve timely and affordable access, and achieve global equity in neurosurgical care.

CLINICS CARE POINTS

- Low and middle income countries bear a disproportionate burden of neurosurgical conditions.
- Clinical missions should incorporate education and training and capacity building to enhance its effectiveness.
- Establishing sustainable partnerships remains an integral part of the field of global neurosurgery.

DISCLOSURE

The authors have no conflict of interest to disclose.

REFERENCES

1. Farmer PE, Kim JY. Surgery and global health: a view from beyond the OR. World J Surg 2008; 32(4):533–6.
2. Meara JG, Leather AJ, Hagander L, et al. Global Surgery 2030: evidence and solutions for achieving health, welfare, and economic development. Lancet (London, England) 2015;386(9993).
3. Unanimously Adopting Historic Sustainable Development Goals. General assembly shapes global outlook for prosperity, Peace | UN Press. Available at: https://press.un.org/en/2015/ga11688.doc.htm. [Accessed 7 October 2023].
4. Kim JY. Opening remarks by Jim Kim, president of the World Bank, to the inaugural meeting of the Lancet commission on global surgery. Boston: Lancet Commission on Global Surgery; 2014. Available at: https://www.youtube.com/watch?v=61iM4Qjk-q4. [Accessed 7 October 2023].
5. World Health Organization. WHA68.15. Strengthening emergency and essential surgical care and anaesthesia as a component of universal health coverage. Available at: https://apps.who.int/gb/ebwha/pdf_files/WHA68/A68_R15-en.pdf. [Accessed 7 October 2023].
6. Dare AJ, Grimes CE, Gillies R, et al. Global surgery: defining an emerging global health field. Lancet (London, England) 2014;384(9961):2245–7.
7. Fuller AT, Barkley A, Du R, et al. Global neurosurgery: a scoping review detailing the current state of international neurosurgical outreach. J Neurosurg 2020; 134(3):1316–24.
8. Dewan MC, Rattani A, Fieggen G, et al. Global neurosurgery: the current capacity and deficit in the provision of essential neurosurgical care. Executive Summary of the Global Neurosurgery Initiative at the Program in Global Surgery and Social Change. J Neurosurg 2018 2018.
9. Park KB, Johnson WD, Dempsey RJ. Global Neurosurgery: The Unmet Need. World Neurosurgery 2016;88:32–5.
10. Mendoza J, Pangal DJ, Cardinal T, et al. Systematic Review of Racial, Socioeconomic, and Insurance Status Disparities in Neurosurgical Care for Intracranial Tumors. World Neurosurg 2021;158: 38–64.
11. Haizel-Cobbina J, Spector LG, Moertel C, et al. Racial and ethnic disparities in survival of children with brain and central nervous tumors in the United States. Pediatr Blood Cancer 2021;68(1):e28738.
12. Chien LC, Wu JC, Chen YC, et al. Age, sex, and socio-economic status affect the incidence of pediatric spinal cord injury: an eleven-year national cohort study. PLoS One 2012;7(6):e39264.
13. Tosoni A, Gatto L, Franceschi E, et al. Association between socioeconomic status and survival in glioblastoma: An Italian single-centre prospective observational study. Eur J Cancer 2021;145:171–8.
14. Servadei F, Rossini Z, Nicolosi F, et al. The Role of Neurosurgery in Countries with Limited Facilities: Facts and Challenges. World Neurosurgery 2018; 112:315–21.
15. Mathers CD, Loncar D. Projections of global mortality and burden of disease from 2002 to 2030. PLoS Med 2006;3(11):e442.
16. Kumar R, Lim J, Mekary RA, et al. Traumatic Spinal Injury: Global Epidemiology and Worldwide Volume. World Neurosurgery 2018;113:e345–63.
17. Rubiano AM, Carney N, Chesnut R, et al. Global neurotrauma research challenges and opportunities. Nature 2015;527(7578):S193–7.
18. Singh G, Sander JW. The global burden of epilepsy report: Implications for low- and middle-income countries. Epilepsy Behav 2020;105:106949.
19. Roach JT, Baticulon RE, Campos DA, et al. The role of neurosurgery in advancing pediatric CNS tumor care worldwide. Brain & Spine 2023;3:101748.
20. Shah SC, Kayamba V, Peek RM, et al. Cancer Control in Low- and Middle-Income Countries: Is It Time to Consider Screening? Journal of Global Oncology 2019;5:1–8.
21. Dewan MC, Rattani A, Mekary R, et al. Global hydrocephalus epidemiology and incidence: systematic review and meta-analysis. J Neurosurg 2018 2018; 130:1065–79.
22. Atta CA, Fiest KM, Frolkis AD, et al. Global Birth Prevalence of Spina Bifida by Folic Acid Fortification Status: A Systematic Review and Meta-Analysis. Am J Publ Health 2016;106(1):e24–34.

23. Dewan MC, Baticulon RE, Rattani A, et al. Pediatric neurosurgical workforce, access to care, equipment and training needs worldwide. Neurosurg Focus 2018;45(4):E13.
24. Mukhopadhyay S, Punchak M, Rattani A, et al. The global neurosurgical workforce: a mixed-methods assessment of density and growth. J Neurosurg 2019 2019;130:1142–8.
25. Haizel-Cobbina J, Chen JW, Belete A, et al. The landscape of neuro-oncology in East Africa: a review of published records. Child's Nerv Syst 2021;37(10):2983–92.
26. Pattisapu JV, Veerappan VR, White C, et al. Spina bifida management in low- and middle-income countries - a comprehensive policy approach. Child's Nerv Syst : CHNS (Child's Nerv Syst) 2023;39(7):1821–9.
27. Sader E, Yee P, Hodaie M. Assessing Barriers to Neurosurgical Care in Sub-Saharan Africa: The Role of Resources and Infrastructure. World Neurosurgery 2017;98:682–8.e3.
28. Kalangu KK. Pediatric neurosurgery in Africa–present and future. Child's Nerv Syst : CHNS (Child's Nerv Syst) 2000;16(10–11):770–5.
29. Ablin G, Fairholm DJ, Kelly DF. Report of FIENS activities. Foundation for International Education in Neurological Surgery. J Neurosurg 1999;90(5):986–7.
30. Ukachukwu AK, Seas A, Petitt Z, et al. Assessing the Success and Sustainability of Global Neurosurgery Collaborations: Systematic Review and Adaptation of the Framework for Assessment of InteRNational Surgical Success Criteria. World Neurosurgery 2022;167:111–21.
31. Lu Z, Tshimbombu TN, Abu-Bonsrah N, et al. Transnational Capacity Building Efforts in Global Neurosurgery: A Review and Analysis of Their Impact and Determinants of Success. World neurosurgery 2023;173:188–98.e3.
32. Bankole NDA, Ouahabi AE. Towards a collaborative-integrative model of education and training in neurosurgery in low and middle-income countries. Clin Neurol Neurosurg 2022;220:107376.
33. Neurosurgical Equipment Support by WFNS. Available at: https://wfns.org/menu/21/neurosurgical-equipment-support. [Accessed 8 October 2023].
34. Fuller A, Tran T, Muhumuza M, et al. Building neurosurgical capacity in low and middle income countries. eNeurologicalSci 2015;3:1–6.
35. Sichimba D, Bandyopadhyay S, Ciuculete AC, et al. Neurosurgical Equipment Donations: A Qualitative Study. Frontiers in Surgery 2022;8:690910.
36. Venturini S, Park KB. Evaluating the Effectiveness and the Impact of Donated Neurosurgical Equipment on Neurosurgical Units in Low- and Middle-Income Countries: The World Federation of Neurosurgical Societies Experience. World Neurosurgery 2018;109:98–109.
37. Adeloye A. Use of the Malawi shunt in the treatment of obstructive hydrocephalus in children. East Afr Med J 1997;74(4):263–6.
38. Chhabra DK. The saga of the 'Chhabra' shunt. Neurol India 2019;67(3):635–8.
39. Warf BC. Comparison of endoscopic third ventriculostomy alone and combined with choroid plexus cauterization in infants younger than 1 year of age: a prospective study in 550 African children. J Neurosurg 2005;103(6 Suppl):475–81.
40. Warf BC. Hydrocephalus in Uganda: the predominance of infectious origin and primary management with endoscopic third ventriculostomy. J Neurosurg 2005;102(1 Suppl).
41. Warf BC, Campbell JW. Combined endoscopic third ventriculostomy and choroid plexus cauterization as primary treatment of hydrocephalus for infants with myelomeningocele: long-term results of a prospective intent-to-treat study in 115 East African infants. J Neurosurg Pediatr 2008;2(5):310–6.
42. Labuschagne J, Mutyaba D, Ouma J, et al. Flexible endoscope-assisted suture release and barrel stave osteotomy for the correction of sagittal synostosis. J Neurosurg Pediatr 2022;31(1):71–7.
43. Robertson FC, Esene IN, Kolias AG, et al. Global Perspectives on Task Shifting and Task Sharing in Neurosurgery. World Neurosurgery 2019;6:100060.
44. Robertson FC, Esene IN, Kolias AG, et al. Task-Shifting and Task-Sharing in Neurosurgery: An International Survey of Current Practices in Low- and Middle-Income Countries. World Neurosurgery 2019;6:100059.
45. Figaji A, Taylor A, Mahmud MR, et al. On progress in Africa, by African experts. Lancet Neurol 2018;17(2):114.
46. Onyia CU, Ojo OA. Collaborative International Neurosurgery Education for Africa-The Journey So Far and the Way Forward. World neurosurgery 2020;141:e566–75.
47. Liang KE, Bernstein I, Kato Y, et al. Enhancing Neurosurgical Education in Low- and Middle-income Countries: Current Methods and New Advances. Neurol Med -Chir 2016;56(11):709–15.
48. Dada OE, Haizel-Cobbina J, Ohonba E, et al. Barriers Encountered Toward Pursuing a Neurosurgical Career: A Cross-Sectional Study Among Medical Students, Interns, and Junior Doctors in Africa. World neurosurgery 2022;166:e388–403.
49. Neurotrauma And Global Neurosurgery International Fellowship. Available at: https://www.globalneurotraumafellowship.com. [Accessed 8 October 2023].
50. Almeida JP, Velásquez C, Karekezi C, et al. Global neurosurgery: models for international surgical education and collaboration at one university. Neurosurg Focus 2018;45(4):E5.
51. de Mello PA. Neurosurgical training in Brazil. World neurosurgery 2012;77(3–4):422–4.

52. World Federation of Neurosurgical Societies WFNS. Training Centers & Guideline | World Federation of Neurosurgical Societies.

53. Madjid Samii. Africa100. JGNS 2021;1(1). Available at: https://journalofglobalneurosurgery.net/index.php/jgns/article/view/5.

54. Kanmounye US, Shlobin NA, Dempsey RJ, et al. Foundation for International Education in Neurosurgery: The Next Half-Century of Service Through Education. JGNS 2021;1(1). Available at: https://journalofglobal neurosurgery.net/index.php/jgns/article/view/28.

55. Rallo MS, Strong MJ, Teton ZE, et al. Targeted Public Health Training for Neurosurgeons: An Essential Task for the Prioritization of Neurosurgery in the Evolving Global Health Landscape. Neurosurgery 2023;92(1):10–7.

56. Lepard JR, Barthélemy EJ, Corley J, et al. The Resident's Role in Global Neurosurgery. World neurosurgery 2020;140. https://doi.org/10.1016/j.wneu.2020.06.004.

57. FIENS. Bootcamps. Available at: https://fiens.org/education/bootcamps/.

58. Hoffman C, Härtl R, Shlobin NA, et al. Future Directions for Global Clinical Neurosurgical Training: Challenges and Opportunities. World neurosurgery 2022;166:e404–18.

59. Warf BC. Educate one to save a few. Educate a few to save many. World neurosurgery 2013;79(2 Suppl): S15.e15–8.

60. Haji FA, Lepard JR, Davis MC, et al. A model for global surgical training and capacity development: the Children's of Alabama-Viet Nam pediatric neurosurgery partnership. Child's Nerv Syst : CHNS (Child's Nerv Syst) 2021;37(2):627–36.

61. Nicolosi F, Rossini Z, Zaed I, et al. Neurosurgical digital teaching in low-middle income countries: beyond the frontiers of traditional education. Neurosurg Focus 2018;45(4):E17.

62. Zuckerman SL, Chanbour H, Haizel-Cobbina J, et al. Neurosurgery Residency Education in the Post-COVID-19 Era: Planning for the Future. World Neurosurgery 2022;158:312–3.

63. The Neurosurgical Atlas. Aaron Cohen-Gadol, M.D. @AaronCohenGadol. Available at: https://www.neurosurgicalatlas.com/. [Accessed 8 October 2023].

64. The Rhoton Collection (2D). Available at: https://www.youtube.com/playlist?list=PL6307C9E54B56AD87. [Accessed 8 October 2023].

65. Interactive Brain Model. BrainFacts.org. Available at: https://www.brainfacts.org:443/3d-brain. [Accessed 8 October 2023].

66. Available at: https://www.upsurgeon.com/. [Accessed 8 October 2023].

67. Brainbook. Available at: https://brainbookcharity.org/. [Accessed 8 October 2023].

68. Touch Surgery. Available at: https://touchsurgery.com. [Accessed 8 October 2023].

69. The ISPN Guide to Pediatric Neurosurgery. Available at: https://ispn.guide/. [Accessed 8 October 2023].

70. Lepard JR, Akbari SHA, Haji F, et al. The initial experience of InterSurgeon: an online platform to facilitate global neurosurgical partnerships. Neurosurg Focus 2020;48(3):E15.

71. Maleknia P, Shlobin NA, Johnston JM, et al. Establishing collaborations in global neurosurgery: The role of InterSurgeon. J Clin Neurosci 2022;100:164–8.

72. Davis MC, Can DD, Pindrik J, et al. Virtual Interactive Presence in Global Surgical Education: International Collaboration Through Augmented Reality. World Neurosurgery 2016;86:103–11.

73. Kubben P. NeuroMind 2: Interactive decision support for neurosurgery. Surg Neurol Int 2012; 3(109).

74. Henderson F, Lepard J, Seibly J, et al. An online tumor board with international neurosurgical collaboration guides surgical decision-making in Western Kenya. Child's Nerv Syst 2021 2021;37(2):715–9.

75. Genomet. @genomet_com. Available at: https://genomet.com/. [Accessed 8 October 2023].

76. FIENS. Virtual Visiting Professor. Available at: https://fiens.org/categories/virtual-visiting-professor/.

77. Haizel-Cobbina J, Thakkar R, Still M, et al. Global Epidemiology of Pediatric Traumatic Spine Injury: A Systematic Review and Meta-Analysis. World Neurosurgery 2023;178:172–80.e3.

78. Paradie E, Warman PI, Waguia-Kouam R, et al. The Scope, Growth, and Inequities of the Global Neurosurgery Literature: A Bibliometric Analysis. World Neurosurgery 2022 2022;167:e670–84.

79. Tropeano MP, Spaggiari R, Ileyassoff H, et al. A comparison of publication to TBI burden ratio of low- and middle-income countries versus high-income countries: how can we improve worldwide care of TBI? Neurosurg Focus 2019;47(5):E5.

80. Vaughan KA, Lopez Ramos C, Buch VP, et al. An estimation of global volume of surgically treatable epilepsy based on a systematic review and meta-analysis of epilepsy. J Neurosurg 2018;130(4):1127–41.

81. Servadei F, Tropeano MP, Spaggiari R, et al. Footprint of Reports From Low- and Low- to Middle-Income Countries in the Neurosurgical Data: A Study From 2015 to 2017. World Neurosurgery 2019;130:e822–30.

82. Kanmounye US, Karekezi C, Nyalundja AD, et al. Adult brain tumors in Sub-Saharan Africa: A scoping review. Neuro Oncol 2022;24(10):1799–806.

83. Griswold DP, Khan AA, Chao TE, et al. Neurosurgical Randomized Trials in Low- and Middle-Income Countries. Neurosurgery 2020;87(3):476–83.

84. Omar AT, Chan KIP, Ong EP, et al. Neurosurgical research in Southeast Asia: A bibliometric analysis. J Clin Neurosci 2022;106:159–65.

85. Program in Global Surgery and Social Change | Harvard Medical School. Available at: https://www.pgssc.org. [Accessed 8 October 2023].

86. National Institutes of Health Fogarty Global Health Training Program for Fellows and Scholars. Available at: https://www.ncbi.nlm.nih.gov/pubmed/. [Accessed 8 October 2023].

87. Clark D, Joannides A, Adeleye AO, et al. Casemix, management, and mortality of patients rreseceiving emergency neurosurgery for traumatic brain injury in the Global Neurotrauma Outcomes Study: a prospective observational cohort study. Lancet Neurol 2022;21(5):438–49.

88. SNOSSA. Available at: https://snossa.org/. [Accessed 8 October 2023].

89. Kanmounye US, Zolo Y, Nguembu S, et al. Training the Next Generation of Academic Global Neurosurgeons: Experience of the Association of Future African Neurosurgeons. Frontiers in surgery 2021;8:631912.

90. Rosseau G, Johnson WD, Park KB, et al. Global neurosurgery: continued momentum at the 72nd World Health Assembly. J Neurosurg 2020;132(4):1256–60.

91. Kancherla V, Botto LD, Rowe LA, et al. Preventing birth defects, saving lives, and promoting health equity: an urgent call to action for universal mandatory food fortification with folic acid. Lancet Global Health 2022;10(7):e1053–7.

92. The Global Surgery Foundation. The NSOAP Manual. Available at: https://www.globalsurgeryfoundation.org/nsoap-manual-program. [Accessed 8 October 2023].

93. El-Ghandour NMF. Neurosurgical education in Egypt and Africa. Neurosurg Focus 2020;48(3):E12.

94. M Selveindran S, Khan MM, Simadibrata DM, et al. Mapping global evidence on strategies and interventions in neurotrauma and road traffic collisions prevention: a scoping review protocol. BMJ Open 2019;9(11):e031517.

95. Rehman AU, Ahmed A, Zaheer Z, et al. International Neurosurgery: The Role for Collaboration. International journal of medical and pharmaceutical research 2023;4(1):15–24.

The Role of Policy in Global Neurosurgery

Faith C. Robertson, MD, MSc, MBA[a,b,*], Kee B. Park, MD, MPH[c],
Walter D. Johnson, MD, MPH, MBA[d,e]

KEYWORDS

- Global neurosurgery • Global health policy • Policy • Guidelines • Advocacy • NSOAP
- National health plan

KEY POINTS

- Global neurosurgery is defined as the clinical and public health practice of neurosurgery with the primary purpose of ensuring timely, safe, and affordable neurosurgical care to all who need it. The public health practice includes informing policies that affect the neurosurgical disease management at the population level.
- National and international policies establish actions to achieve stated goals. They also facilitate cooperation among nations to align on universal measures and objectives to implement sustainable solutions.
- Comprehensive disease management encompasses surveillance, prevention, pre-hospital care, hospital care, and rehabilitation services. Furthermore, the approach is systematic by addressing the 6 building blocks of the health system (1) Infrastructure; (2) Workforce; (3) Service delivery; (4) Financing; (5) Information management; and (6) Governance.
- Examples of recent collaborative policy recommendations include those for Head and Spine Injury Care as well as Management of Spina Bifida and Hydrocephalus in Low-income and Middle-income Countries.
- Continued research is needed to inform future policies, and advocacy thereafter is instrumental in ensuring sustainable improvement in neurosurgical care globally.

INTRODUCTION

The global neurosurgery movement emerged with increasing recognition of the impact of neurologic disorders on public health, and of neurosurgery as an integral part of global health systems improvement. Each year, over 5 million people with neurosurgical conditions do not receive the essential treatment required, with the greatest inequities occurring in low-income and middle-income countries (LMICs).[1] This disparity propagates morbidity, mortality, and economic losses.[2] Global neurosurgery as a field is defined as the clinical and public health practice of neurosurgery with the primary purpose of ensuring timely, safe, and affordable neurosurgical care to all who need it. It includes the practice, study, and advocacy of neurosurgery on a global scale, including efforts to address access to neurosurgical care and resources across different regions and countries. A cardinal element in driving sustainable change is engaging in policy dialogue as content experts.

Multinational political commitment, such as the World Health Assembly (WHA) resolutions, facilitates cooperation among nations to align on universal measures and objectives to implement

[a] Department of Neurosurgery, Massachusetts General Hospital, Boston, MA, USA; [b] Harvard Business School, Boston, MA, USA; [c] Global Neurosurgery Initiative, Program in Global Surgery and Social Change, Harvard Medical School, Boston, MA, USA; [d] Department of Neurosurgery, Loma Linda University, CA, USA; [e] Mercy Ships, Garden Valley, TX, USA
* Corresponding author. Massachusetts General Hospital, Harvard Medical School, Room Gray 502, 55 Fruit Street, Boston, MA.
E-mail address: frobertson@mgh.harvard.edu

Neurosurg Clin N Am 35 (2024) 401–410
https://doi.org/10.1016/j.nec.2024.05.002
1042-3680/24/© 2024 Elsevier Inc. All rights are reserved, including those for text and data mining, AI training, and similar technologies.

sustainable solutions. Global neurosurgery practitioners can contribute to the process by generating accurate assessment of the burden of neurosurgical disease, identifying areas of improvement, and recommend interventions. Policies that recognize the importance of neurosurgical services within broader health agendas can lead to increased funding, training programs, and infrastructure development that ultimately benefit the population by improving neurosurgical outcomes.

Global efforts to improve surgical care, including neurosurgical care has seen significant policy milestones and landmarks over the past decade, from the Lancet Commission on Global Surgery and the Bogotá Declaration to the development and adoption of National Obstetric, Anesthesia, and Surgical Plans (NSOAPs) that integrate neurosurgery into broader health care frameworks and contribute to improved policy development and resource allocation.

In this article, we will highlight key historic policy milestones in the global neurosurgery movement. We will discuss the role of international organizations in neurosurgery, and the incorporation of neurosurgery into global health agendas. We will then delve into specific examples of international and national policies that have been established, highlight the role of international organizations in shaping neurosurgical policies, emphasize the importance of advocacy, and explore future directions.

HISTORICAL BACKGROUND

While efforts to enhance the level of neurosurgical care globally have existed for many years, only recently did the field of global neurosurgery become more formalized and aligned at scale. **Fig. 1** is not a fully comprehensive timeline, but highlights key moments in that evolution, beginning a rapid succession of events in 2015. First, the

Sustainable Development Goals (SDGs) for 2030 set by the United Nations included many more topics relevant to surgical care than the Millennium Development Goals, going from 8 goals with 18 targets to 17 goals with 169 targets.[3] The 3rd Edition of the Disease Control Priorities (DCP-3) report included Volume 1 on Essential Surgery, which identified 44 surgical procedures as essential on the basis that they address substantial needs, are cost effective, and are feasible to implement.[4] The Lancet Commission on Global Surgery in 2015 further emphasized that surgery is an integral, indivisible component of a properly functioning health system.[2] It leveraged data from multiple foundational papers to support that investing in surgical services in LMICs is affordable, saves lives, and promotes economic growth, and was necessary to achieve the SDGs. Metrics from the Lancet Commission included access to timely essential surgery, specialist workforce density, surgical volume, perioperative mortality, and protection against impoverishing and catastrophic expenditure. Striking results from that assessment included that 143 million additional surgical procedures are needed in LMICs each year to save lives and prevent disability, and only 6% of the procedures at that time were occurring in the poorest countries, where one-third of the world population lived. Additionally, the 2015 WHA Resolution 68.15 was wholly focused on strengthening emergency and essential surgical care and anesthesia as a necessary part of universal health coverage.[5] These 4 events, which occurred in rapid succession, catapulted global surgical care into the spotlight and served as a call to action to address surgery on the global political agenda.

To guide development of sustainable surgical systems, the Harvard's Program of Global Surgery and Social Change (PGSSC) partnered with several Ministries of Health to develop NSOAPs that are

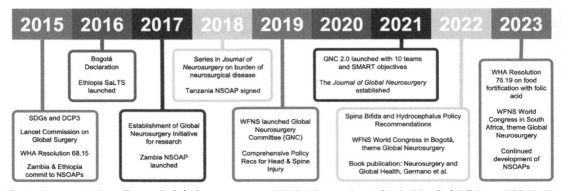

Fig. 1. Key events in policy and global neurosurgery. DCP3, Disease Control Priorities 3rd Editions; NSOAP, National Surgical, Obstetric and Anesthesia plans; SaLTS, Saving Lives Through Safe Surgery; SDGs, Sustainable Development Goals.

fully embedded within the national health policy, strategy, or plan. The process of NSOAP development is specific to each country and elucidates current gaps in health care, prioritizes solutions, and provides specific time bound, prioritized implementation plans.[6] It includes: (1) Infrastructure; (2) Workforce; (3) Service delivery; (4) Financing; (5) Information management; and (6) Governance. By working with governments to foster new policies that incorporate these 6 building blocks, context-specific plans could be made that aligned on universal measures and objectives, garnered appropriate financial and human resource involvement, and laid the groundwork to implement sustainable solutions. Zambia and Ethiopia were 2 of the first countries to commit to national strategies for improving surgical and anesthesia care in 2015, and will be discussed further in this chapter.

Neurosurgery is an important subspecialty to involve in health system strengthening given the disease burden and cost-effectiveness.[1,7] Each year, an estimated 22.6 million patients suffer from neurologic disorders or injuries that warrant a neurosurgical evaluation, and of these, 13.8 million individuals would require surgery. Unfortunately, approximately 5 million essential neurosurgical cases go untreated, and over 23,000 more neurosurgeons are needed in LMICs to address this treatment gap; this number is projected to increase rapidly over the next 2 to 3 decades.[8] For instance, stroke mortality and daily adjusted life years lost are expected to rise from around 7 million to 10 million, and 45 million to 190 million (respectively) by 2050; as hemorrhagic stroke rates in LMIC are at minimum 34%, this has significant implications for both endovascular and open neurosurgery.[9] Furthermore, of the 17 SDGs for 2030, 14 require building surgical capacity and have direct or indirect relevance to neurosurgeons and neurosurgical care delivery.[10] The DCP-3 Vol 1 Essential Surgery indicated that district hospitals should be able to perform burr holes for hematomas and elevated intracranial pressure and shunts for hydrocephalus, while tertiary care centers should have the capacity to perform craniotomies and craniectomies, predominantly for neurotrauma.[4] However, current resource limitations and neurosurgical workforce deficits continue to be significant barriers to such care provision.[1]

Consequently, in december 2016, leaders of organized neurosurgery met during the International Conference on Recent Advances in Neurotraumatology in Bogotá, Colombia to recognize the tremendous deficit in global neurosurgical care and simultaneously call on our own professional community to unite and play a leading role as agents for change. The 2016 Bogotá Declaration

the first document of its kind and was a significant landmark in catalyzing the rise of national and international policies positioned to tackle the global burden of neurosurgical disease.[11]

As you cannot manage what you do not measure, this spurred additional transnational collaborations in research in burden of disease and gaps in access to care. It also sparked the launch of the Global Neurosurgery Initiative at the PGSSC to galvanize additional investigations and coalesce data into policy recommendations. In 2018, the Journal of Neurosurgery released a series of publications from this group that articulated the burden of disease as it related to traumatic brain injury, hydrocephalus, infection, epilepsy, oncology, and more. It also quantified the geographic operative and consultation demands, workforce need, and examined academic collaborations. These findings were incorporated into the "Comprehensive Policy Recommendations for Head and Spine Injury Care in Low-Income and Middle-Income Countries" in 2019, and the "Comprehensive Policy Recommendations for the Management of Spina Bifida and Hydrocephalus in Low-Income and Middle-Income Countries" in 2022 (discussed in more detail below).[12,13]

By 2019, 5 countries had completed an NSOAP and an additional 37 member states had either completed or were in the process of drafting or initiating a National Plan for Surgical Care 13. Also in 2019, the World Federation of Neurosurgical Societies (WFNS) established the Global Neurosurgery Committee, which greatly complimented an long-standing the World Health Organisation (WHO)-WFNS Liaison Committee. The aim of this committee is designing a global action plan with 5 key objectives and over 20 targets. The 5 objectives were: (1) Amplify neurosurgical access, (2) Align global neurosurgery activity, (3) Advance relevant research, especially from LMICs, (4) Assimilate global neurosurgery activity within the global surgery framework, and (5) Advocate for neurosurgical care for all.

In 2021, the Global Neuroosurgery Committee (GNC) established its 2.0 plan, with a structure that is decentralized with multiple thematic teams, each with their own strategic plans. The teams are Workforce, Coordination, Research, Policy, Decolonize, External Relations, Capacity Building, Global Spine Surgery, Nursing, Advocacy, Innovation and Technology, Neurodiagnostics, and Young Neurosurgeons. The 10 teams have developed mini-strategic plans with Specific, Measurable, Attainable, Relevant, and Time-based objectives. 2021 also was a landmark year for the launch of the Journal of Global Neurosurgery. This is a free, open access journal that gives preferences to LMIC authors to ensure research in the most affected countries is being empowered and shared.

In 2022, the Spina Bifida and Hydrocephalus Policy Recommendations were released, and a resolution was introduced to the WHA in May 2022 by WFNS in collaboration with the Global Alliance for Prevention of Spina Bifida.[14] This lead to the 2023 adoption of WHA resolution 76.19 calling for mandatory folic acid food fortification along with other micronutrients to combat preventable micronutrient deficiencies, such as spina bifida and neural tube defects.[15] That year, the WFNS World Congress was held in Bogotá with a theme of Global Neurosurgery. Additionally, Springer published a book *Neurosurgery and Global Health,* edited by Dr. Isabelle Germano and authored by many of the content experts in global neurosurgery.[16] In 2023, there were continued global efforts on the development and implementation of NSOAPs and the WFNS World Congress in Cape Town, South Africa with a full day dedicated to global initiatives.

With that overview of the landscape of progress within global neurosurgery, we will delve further into the policy recommendations for Head and Spine Injury as well for the Management of Spina Bifida and Hydrocephalus in LMICs, and then highlight case examples of NSOAPs that have integrated these frameworks into their national policy.

COMPREHENSIVE POLICY RECOMMENDATIONS FOR HEAD AND SPINE INJURY

Head and spine injuries were the initial focus because in LMICs global neurotrauma comprises the highest proportion of unmet neurosurgical operative burden, with almost 5 million cases per year. These policy recommendations were intended to be nested within the NSOAP framework of addressing the 6 domains of a health care system (infrastructure, workforce, service delivery, financing, information management, and governance). The neurotrauma policy recommendations added domains adapted from proposals by the American College of Surgeons for improving trauma systems.[17] This includes: (1) Surveillance; (2) Prevention; (3) Pre-hospital care; (4) Surgical system; and (5) Rehabilitation. Herein, the policy recommendations create a matrix across the 6 domains of health care (**Fig. 2**).

Within the document, each frame of the matrix is supported with data and includes principles for guidance for the policy maker. For example, under *Surveillance*, there is guidance on establishing a neurotrauma registry including more granular recommendations on minimum data to include relating to demographics, diagnosis, mechanism, severity, and outcome measures. It discusses how the WHO Trauma System Maturity Index and the WHO International Registry for Trauma and Emergency Care can be leveraged to achieve national surveillance. There are recommendations for sources of funding and collaboration to meet the financial burden associated with establishing these networks, as well as guidance on involving medical associations in legislative and government processes for the development and organization of an effective trauma registry.

Under *Prevention*, the document goes beyond foundational elements of safe roads. It gives evidence for revisiting the national and local laws, such as those on helmets. The document also highlights logistical and cultural barriers that may be at play in law enforcement. For example, Bachani and colleagues found the rate of helmet usage among motorbike riders in Cambodia to be as low as 33% 3 years after the passage of helmet legislation, with misconceptions from riders that they are unnecessary for short distance or at low speeds.[18] Additionally, the document references a study in Vietnam that found a primary reason for adults not having young children wear helmets was secondary to fear that it increases the risk of neck injury.[19] Thus, it describes how effective injury prevention strategy must include public education and media campaigns to increase compliance.

Overall, this policy document provides both a compass and a roadmap for policy leaders to integrate local laws, campaigns, research, and change efforts into their local health ecosystem.

COMPREHENSIVE POLICY RECOMMENDATIONS FOR THE MANAGEMENT OF SPINA BIFIDA AND HYDROCEPHALUS

The subsequent comprehensive policy recommendation effort mirrored that of the neurotrauma recommendations above. It was guided by the PGSSC as well as an international expert advisory group. An international group consisting of neurologists, pediatricians, neurosurgeons, surgeons, anesthesiologists, and nurses, as well as professional societies, patient advocates, researchers, global health practitioners, and policy makers from 18 countries and 4 continents. The recommendations were divided into the following sections: (1) screening and surveillance, (2) prevention, (3) pre-hospital care, (4) surgical systems, (5) rehabilitation, and (6) transitional and follow-up care (**Fig. 3**). The authors recognize that the data and recommendations are intentioned to serve as a starting point to

	Surveillance	Prevention	Pre-hospital care	Surgical system	Rehabilitation
Infra-structure	-Integration through agile platforms -Leverage international partnerships for surveillance	-Safe roads	-Contextualized pre-hospital system	-80% of population within 4-hours of neurotrauma center -Strengthen pre-existing trauma infrastructure for neurotrauma	-Contextualized allocation of space and stuff for neuro-rehabilitation -Facility stratification for severity
Workforce	-Fit for purpose workforce for data collection, analysis, and interpretation -Align international collaborations to support local workforce capacity - Flexible and strategic use task-shifting and task-sharing to optimize human resources	-Robust workforce for public health education and implementation	-Neurotrauma care training of emergency medical personnel	-1 neurosurgeon per 200,000 people at minimum -Task-sharing of surgical workforce is preferred over task-shifting -Dramatically increase neurosurgical training capacity	-Ensure rehabilitation training capacity is adequate -Ensure competency throughout continuum education
Service delivery	-Minimum data to include demographics, diagnosis, mechanism, severity, and outcome measure -Use existing trauma registry -Use WHO Trauma System Maturity Index to monitor progress	-Strengthen public education -Encourage safety-conscious "Ride hailing" services -Strengthen enforcement of safety laws	-Prevent hypotension and maintain oxygenation -Time from injury to neurotrauma facility should not exceed 4-hours	-Standardization of essential neurotrauma equipment -CT scanner in all neurotrauma facilities -Critical care unit in all neurotrauma facilities -Leverage telemedicine as a tool for increasing coverage - Innovate for low-resource settings	-Sensitive to gender and age sub-groups - Partner with family for delivery of non-technical physical therapy
Financing	-Maximize external funding -Build internal capacity -Use open-source platforms	-Promote health benefits of public investment in safe roads -Partner with external organizations for advocacy	-Cost-effective training models -Utilize low-cost or free digital technology	-Embed neurotrauma within universal health coverage package -International partnerships for neurotrauma capacity building	-Embed neurorehabilitation within universal health coverage package
Information management	-Utilize WHO International Registry for Trauma and Emergency Care (IRTEC)	-Tracking of safety law compliance	-Encourage data collection by emergency medical personnel	-Track neurotrauma workforce and operative mortality	-Collection of neurorehabilitation outcome data
Governance	-Empower ministry of health leadership -Utilize reporting requirements to improve accountability and compliance	-Regulatory framework to strengthen enforcement -Comprehensive helmet laws - Workplace safety regulations	-Inclusion of pre-hospital care in national health plans	-Draw on existing international technical resources to assist with neurotrauma capacity building -Promote neurotrauma as vital to achieving national and international health and development goals	-Rehabilitation is indispensable to a quality health system

Fig. 2. Head and spine injury recommendations matrix. (Published by Park, Khan and colleagues, 2019.[12])

engage the patients, health care providers, public health practitioners, and policymakers in a productive dialogue that will lead to smart policies and tangible outcomes for children with spina bifida and hydrocephalus in LMICs.

CASE STUDIES OF SUCCESSFUL INTEGRATION OF NEUROSURGERY INTO NATIONAL HEALTH POLICIES
Ethiopia

With the momentum of the 2015 Lancet Commission on Global Surgery, Ethiopia was one of the first countries to pledge intention to develop a systematic national strategy. In 2016, they released the Federal Ministry of Health of Ethiopia National Safe Surgery Strategic PLAN: Saving Lives Through Safe Surgery (SaLTS) with a timeframe of 2016 to 2020.[20] At the start, the WFNS workforce density map showed Ethiopia with a density of neurosurgeons of 0.025 per 100,000 populations to reflect the 25 neurosurgeons for a population of 97 million people, ranking them 150th in the world.[21] Ethiopia was actively working to scale their neurosurgery workforce, as they reflected on the striking statistical of only having 2 neurosurgeons who cared for the entire population in 2006.[22] In the SaLTS plan, the government set a goal of achieving a workforce of 50 neurosurgeons by 2020, which they indeed achieved with 50 attending neurosurgeons and 80 neurosurgical residents, putting the neurosurgeon density per 100,000 people at 0.045. The growth rate for the number of neurosurgeons and neurosurgery residents was 20% and 26.3%, respectively,

	Surveillance	Prevention	Prehospital Care	Surgical Care	Rehabilitation	Transitional Care
Infrastructure	-Head circumference measurements -Common data elements -Improve access to obstetric facilities	-Neonatal sepsis treatment -Microbial diagnostics -Folic acid supplementation	-WHO Emergency Care System -Strengthen multisectoral coordination	-Strengthen Surgical System -80% population coverage -Expand first-level hospitals	-Designated rehabilitation space -Disabled-friendly infrastructure	-National strategy for life-long care -Community-based rehabilitation -People-centered facilities
Workforce	-Use non-physician workforce -Train parents/caregivers - Destigmatize	-Increase prenatal care workforce -Family involvement -Advocacy groups	-Education of care team -Support families	-Increase pediatric providers -Dedicated training centers. -Task shifting/sharing	-Training and education -Task sharing/task shifting	-Patient empowerment -Coordination by nurses and CHW
Service Delivery	-Community-based screening -Public health education -Universal databases	-Parental education -Folic acid fortification -Public education	-Public health campaigns -Coordinate dispatch	-Multidisciplinary teams - Wards for SB/HCP patients - Access to imaging	-Multidisciplinary care teams -Engage family/caregivers in rehabilitation care	-Safe transition to adulthood
Financing	-Government funding - NGO funding -Leverage international partnerships	-Fund infant care -Fund Folic acid supplementation -Funding education	Affordable transportation	-Include SB/HCP care into UHC -Consider international partnerships	Embed into a UHC package	Embed in UHC
Information Management	-National registries -WSeb-based platforms -Standardization	-National registries. -Common data elements	-Optimize referrals -Strengthen data collection	-Track SB/HCP workforce	Rehabilitation data	- Quality of life metrics -Health Passport model
Governance	-Screening & reporting mandate -Support to the Ministry of Health	-Child health legislation -Folic Acid legislation -National Prevention Campaign	-Emergency service teams -Disability rights legislation	Dedicated SB/HCP teams	Establish departments	-Protect rights of SB/HCP patients -Multidisciplinary Transition teams

Fig. 3. Comprehensive policy recommendations for the management of spina bifida and hydrocephalus.

from 2006 to 2020. In a 2021 article by Asfaw and colleagues entitled *Neurosurgery in Ethiopia: A New Chapter and Future Prospects,* the authors reflect on this journal and future directions. To achieve such growth, Ethiopia forged international partnership between the Addis Ababa University, University of Bergen, Haukel and the University Hospital, and a private hospital in Addis Ababa. Other institutions such as the U.S-based Foundation for International Education in Neurologic Surgery (FIENS) contributed to the success of the partnership by arranging for dedicated volunteer neurosurgeons to stay in Addis Ababa from weeks to months and teach resident physicians. They also placed a tremendous emphasis on developing local research capacity; greater than 77% of the neurosurgical publications pertinent to Ethiopia were published since the first class of residents graduated in 2010.

Importantly, Asfaw and colleagues also frames the tremendous progress in the context of recent policy recommendations. In their reference to the 2019 *Comprehensive Policy Recommendations for Head and Spine Injury,* they underscore that there should be 0.5 neurosurgeon per 100,000 people, making the 560 the minimum number of required neurosurgeons in Ethiopia. However, they are optimistic that if they can sustain a high retention rate for locally trained neurosurgeons coupled with the gradual increase in state resources devoted to surgical development, Ethiopia could achieve this workforce target. Based on growth rates of the total population and neurosurgical workforce, Ethiopia will have a neurosurgeon density greater than 0.5 per 100,000 people by 2036. Their example of a self-sustained neurosurgery program transforms both the clinical capacity and the academic productivity of local neurosurgeons. Overall, the neurosurgical development in Ethiopia demonstrates the profound effect of leveraging policy to formulate benchmarks and secure funding and establish training programs via international partnerships to improve neurosurgical access.

Zambia

The Republic of Zambia, former Minister of Health Dr. Chitalu Chilufya (term: 2016–2021), and Counsellor-Health, Permanent Mission of Zambia to the UN in Geneva, Dr. Emmanuel Makasa (term: 2012–2018) have been champions in efforts to expand access to surgical care, sponsoring and chairing the diplomatic negotiations that culminated in the development and adoption of WHA68.15 in 2015 and subsequently Decision WHA70(22) in 2017 that requires WHO Director-General to report on their progress of WHA68.15 every 2 years.[23]

Zambia was a leader in establishing an NSOAP that proactively spoke to many of the subspecialties as well.[24,25] With respect to neurosurgery, they listed the number of facilities offering neurosurgical services at a base of 1 in 2017, with a goal of 3 in 2019 and 7 by 2021. For the number of facilities offering spinal surgery services, there was a base of 1 in 2017, and a goal of 2 in 2019 and 2021. On workforce, ideal staffing quota for neurosurgeons was 1 neurosurgeon per Level 2 Hospital and 5 neurosurgeons per Level 3 Hospital. They projected this into a framework for evaluation that identified the national need of 70 neurosurgeons and the dramatic deficit of 68 neurosurgeons at that time. To understand the financial requirements involved for this capacity escalation, the team modeled Human Resources Needs and Costing. For Training over the next 5 years focusing on district hospitals, with a 3-year goal of 5 neurosurgeons and a 5-year goal of 12 additional (17 total), accounting for a 4-year training span, the cost per provider per year would be 325,762.50, and 22,151,850.00 in total. This was within the multidisciplinary total workforce training cost of 612,252,925.00 Kwacha ($USD 23,422,966). Having the detailed strategic plan with required resources laid out enables better commitment of funding and prioritization of the efforts. Today, the total number of neurosurgeons in Zambia fluctuates around 90, though not all are Zambian nationals; most are accredited by the College of Surgeons of East, Central, and Southern Africa.

Nigeria

Nigeria's Federal Ministry of Health developed and implemented their second National Strategic Health Development Plan for 2018 to 2022, which would integrate their National Surgical, Obstetrics, Anesthesia, and Nursing Plan (NSOANP) that they formulated in 2017. They named this subdivision of focus Strategic Priorities for Surgical Care (StraPS), which introduced specific surgical system targets and an implementation roadmap that prioritized monitoring, evaluation, and feedback for central and state governments to follow. StraPS was one of the first to include children's surgery in a surgical plan, which is highly relevant in Nigeria given that 43% of the 200 million population is under 15 years of age.[26] They also incorporated scaling nursing workforce in the plan.

Neurosurgery has been addressed in several contexts in Nigeria's NSOANP. While the WHO's recommendation is an ideal ratio for every population to be 1 neurosurgeon to 100,000 individuals, Nigeria currently has 0.01 neurosurgeons per 100,000 (29 neurosurgeons at the time of the document).[6] A publication by Garba (Harvard Medical School), Alfin (Jos University Teaching Hospital, Katon Rikkos, Nigeria), and Mahmud (National Hospital, Abuja, Nigeria) in *Frontiers in Surgery* is an example of leveraging prior policy recommendations to fuel engagement of the neurosurgical community with health care planners and policy makers.[27]

Garba and colleagues call on some specific strengths and areas for improvement in the plan. The NSOANP does cite neural tube defects as priorities of basic surgical care provision, which aligns with the comprehensive spina bifida and hydrocephalus recommendations. Nigeria committed to building the capacity at district and secondary hospitals to handle diagnosis and stabilization of neurologic trauma (eg, epidural hematoma, includes emergency burr hole if transfer not possible). They also prioritized training anesthesia subspecialties in neuro-anesthesia.

To build their workforce, Garba and colleagues suggest that a 2-tiered approach to training can be adopted in order to address the immediate need while working on the long-term strategy to improve the number of trained neurosurgeons in the country. For example, in the spirit of task sharing discussed in the *Comprehensive Policy Recommendations for Head and Spine Injury,* a fast–tracked, competency-based certification of General and Pediatric surgeons who can perform neurotrauma operations and neural tube defect surgeries could be adopted. Secondly, the authors call for an acceleration of neurosurgical training by both the National Post graduate Medical College of Nigeria and the West African College of Surgeon that would allow those interested in neurosurgery to fast-track into specialized training without going through a general surgery training. There is also additional emphasis on the need for a formalized neurotrauma registry.

Both the current national plan in Nigeria as well as the calls to action in the recent publication that are rooted in international policy recommendations are key examples of how policy can provide guidance and a foundation for systems level change.

ROLE OF INTERNATIONAL ORGANIZATIONS IN SHAPING NEUROSURGICAL POLICIES

International organizations play a crucial role in shaping neurosurgical policies globally. Their involvement spans a range of activities, from facilitating research that serves as the foundation for policy development and partnering with governments to craft the NSOAPs, to providing human resources and funding to enable execution of the goals. Key players in the global neurosurgery effort are listed here.

G4 Alliance

The Global Alliance for Surgical, Obstetric, Trauma, and Anesthesia Care is a coalition of over 70 member organizations dedicated to advocating globally for the neglected surgical patient. They work to increase awareness, foster political will, shape policy, and mobilize resources. The G4 Alliance Strategic Plan and Theory of Change for 2022 to 2024 describe their advocacy goals and strategies under 3 pillars: awareness, policy, and resource mobilization. They played a key role in advancing the policy agenda of WHA Resolution 68.15, and continue aiding in the development of national surgical plans.

World Federation of Neurosurgical Societies

WFNS is a professional, scientific, non-governmental organization comprising of 130 member societies and over 30,000 neurosurgeons worldwide. For many years the WFNS has the honored status of a non-State actor in official working relations with the WHO. In 2019, the WFNS established the Global Neurosurgery Committee. The committee developed a definition of global neurosurgery which has been widely adopted–the clinical and public health practice of neurosurgery with the primary purpose of ensuring timely, safe, and affordable neurosurgical care to all who need it. The committee also rolled out the global action plan with the help of the secretariat consisting of medical students and trainees from around the world. The second Global Neurosurgery Committee (2021–2023) created thematic teams to implement mini-strategic plans to achieve their set goals and the results were presented over multiple sessions at the WFNS World Congress in Cape Town in December 2023. The third iteration of the Global Neurosurgery Committee

will seek to support on the ground capacity building in those countries with little or no neurosurgical care capacity such as Sierra Leone through strategic partnerships.

Foundation for International Education in Neurologic Surgery

FIENS is highly involved in capacity-building initiatives. They have partnered with multiple institutions to develop international curricula for training programs, which can be certified LMICs. They work to find the equipment, supplies, and mentoring to allow the development of such programs until they become self-sustaining, further dedicated to the post-graduate education of these individuals.

FUTURE DIRECTIONS

As we have seen, there have been tremendous strides over the past decade to institute strong policy as means to facilitate alignment on goals and strategies for global surgical systems strengthening. These international efforts allow the neurosurgery community to engage with policymakers, governments, and other stakeholders to raise awareness about the importance of neurosurgical services and to influence policies that support health system strengthening and service delivery capacity building at the national level. The establishment of the NSOAP framework has fueled multiple nations to implement their own national objectives on improvement of surgical systems within their broader national health plans. Furthermore, the development of comprehensive recommendations for neurotrauma, spina bifida, and hydrocephalus has furthered the detail to which neurosurgical objectives can be instituted to augment care and mitigate the burden of neurosurgical disease worldwide.

Going forward, we as a neurosurgical community must come together to increase efforts in advocacy, further the recommendations for additional neurosurgical subspecialties and associated technologies, as well as partner with neurosurgical leaders across the globe to form national context-specific plans (NSOAPs). Though, the work does not stop there. Policy helps ensure goal alignment and dedication of funds, but much work must go into policy adoption, implementation, and enforcement. Policy formation also calls the global neurosurgical community to action to assist in resource provision and investment in training, building data registries, developing resource-stratified guidelines for specific neurosurgical conditions through expert teams, enabling research in the local context, regularly examining progress, and sharing knowledge. It is only through the unity of policy makers, practitioners, and researchers that we can raise the level of neurosurgical care throughout the world.

CLINICS CARE POINTS

- Policy helps ensure goal alignment and dedication of funds, but subsequent effort must go into policy adoption, adaptation to the local context, implementation, and enforcement.
- The NSOAP framework can help national governments structure their goals and action steps for improvement of surgical systems within their broader national health plan.

DISCLOSURE

F.C. Robertson has conflicts of interest with the Zeta Surgical Inc. and the Johnson and Johnson, none of which are pertinent to this manuscript. K.B. Park holds advisory shares of Hoth Intelligence.

REFERENCES

1. Dewan MC, Rattani A, Fieggen G, et al. Global neurosurgery: the current capacity and deficit in the provision of essential neurosurgical care. Executive Summary of the Global Neurosurgery Initiative at the Program in Global Surgery and Social Change. J Neurosurg 2018;1–10. https://doi.org/10.3171/2017.11.JNS171500.

2. Meara JG, Leather AJ, Hagander L, et al. Global Surgery 2030: Evidence and solutions for achieving health, welfare, and economic development. Surgery 2015;158(1):3–6. https://doi.org/10.1016/j.surg.2015.04.011.

3. Ahmed F, Michelen S, Massoud R, et al. Are the SDGs leaving safer surgical systems behind? Int J Surg 2016;36(Pt A):74–5. https://doi.org/10.1016/j.ijsu.2016.09.095.

4. Mock CN, Donkor P, Gawande A, et al. Essential surgery: key messages from Disease Control Priorities, 3rd edition. Lancet 2015;385(9983):2209–19. https://doi.org/10.1016/S0140-6736(15)60091-5.

5. WHA. Strengthening emergency and essential surgical care and anaesthesia as a component of universal health coverage. 2015. Available at: http://apps.who.int/gb/ebwha/pdf_files/wha68/a68_r15-en.pdf.

6. PGSSC. National Surgical, Obstetric and Anesthesia Planning. Harvard Program in Global Surgery and Social Change. Available at: https://www.pgssc.org/national-surgical-planning.

7. Rudolfson N, Dewan MC, Park KB, et al. The economic consequences of neurosurgical disease in low- and middle-income countries. J Neurosurg 2018;1–8. https://doi.org/10.3171/2017.12.Jns17281.

8. Dewan MC, Rattani A, Gupta S, et al. Estimating the global incidence of traumatic brain injury. J Neurosurg 2018;1–18. https://doi.org/10.3171/2017.10.Jns17352.

9. Feigin VL, Owolabi MO. Pragmatic solutions to reduce the global burden of stroke: a World Stroke Organization-Lancet Neurology Commission. Lancet Neurol 2023;22(12):1160–206. https://doi.org/10.1016/s1474-4422(23)00277-6.

10. Barthelemy EJ, Park KB, Johnson W. Neurosurgery and Sustainable Development Goals. World Neurosurg 2018;120:143–52. https://doi.org/10.1016/j.wneu.2018.08.070.

11. Park KB, Johnson WD, Dempsey RJ. Global Neurosurgery: The Unmet Need. World Neurosurgery 2016;88:32–5.

12. Park K, Tariq K, Olufemi Adeleye A, et al. Comprehensive Policy Recommendations for Head and Spine Injury Care in LMICs. 2019. Available at: https://docs.wixstatic.com/ugd/d9a674_1ba60c38a07341a7bbbe8b1e3f0ff507.pdf.

13. Comprehensive Policy Recommendations for the Management of Spina Bifida & Hydrocephalus in Low- & Middle-Income Countries. 2021;2(1). Available at: https://usercontent.one/wp/www.chyspr.org/wp-content/uploads/2022/03/SBHC-Policy-Recommendations-Full.pdf?media=1636845685.

14. Kirchner S. Food fortification resolution to prevent spina bifida adopted by World Health Organization at the 76th World Health Assembly. Available at: https://www.uab.edu/news/health/item/13648-food-fortification-resolution-to-prevent-spina-bifida-adopted-by-world-health-organization-at-the-76th-world-health-assembly. [Accessed 28 January 2024].

15. ASSEMBLY. WHOS-SWH. List of decisions and resolutions. 2023. Available at: https://apps.who.int/gb/ebwha/pdf_files/WHA76/A76_DIV3-en.pdf.

16. Germano IM. Neurosurgery and global health. Cham, Switzerland: Springer Nature Switzerland AG; 2022.

17. Committee on Trauma ACoS. Regional Trauma Systems: Optimal Elements, Integration, and Assessment. Systems Consultation Guide 2008;2008.

18. Bachani AM, Branching C, Ear C, et al. Trends in prevalence, knowledge, attitudes, and practices of helmet use in Cambodia: results from a two year study. Injury 2013;44(Suppl 4):S31–7. https://doi.org/10.1016/s0020-1383(13)70210-9.

19. Pervin A, Passmore J, Sidik M, et al. Viet Nam's mandatory motorcycle helmet law and its impact on children. Bull World Health Organ 2009;87(5):369–73. https://doi.org/10.2471/blt.08.057109.

20. Federal Ministry of Health of Ethiopia National Safe Surgery Strategic PLAN: Saving Lives Through Safe Surgery (SaLTS) (2017).

21. Societies TWFoN, Global Neurosurgical Workforce Map, ministry of health policy document, Available at: https://www.moh.gov.et/en/initiatives-4-col/Saving_Lives_Through_Safe_Surgery?language_content_entity=en.

22. Asfaw ZK, Tirsit A, Barthélemy EJ, et al. Neurosurgery in Ethiopia: A New Chapter and Future Prospects. World Neurosurgery 2021;152:e175–83.

23. Organization WH. World Health Assembly Resolution 70(22): Progress in the Implementation of the 2030 Agenda for Sustainable Development. 2017.

24. Health. RoZMo. National surgical, obstetric and anesthesia strategic plan (NSOAP): year 2017–2021. Republic of Zambia Ministry of Health; 2017. Available at: https://apps.who.int/gb/ebwha/pdf_files/WHA70/A70(22)-en.pdf.

25. Mukhopadhyay S, Lin Y, Mwaba P, et al. National surgical, obstetric, and anesthesia strategic plan development–the Zambian experience. ACS Bull 2017;102:6.

26. Peters AW, Roa L, Rwamasirabo E, et al. National Surgical, Obstetric, and Anesthesia Plans Supporting the Vision of Universal Health Coverage. Glob Health Sci Pract 2020;8(1):1–9. https://doi.org/10.9745/ghsp-d-19-00314.

27. Garba DL, Alfin DJ, Mahmud MR. The Incorporation of Neurosurgery as an Integral Part of the Strategic Priorities for Surgical Care in Nigeria. Opinion. Frontiers in Surgery 2021;8:689180.

Neurosurgical Advocacy in the Prevention of Neural Tube Defects

Impacting Global Fortification Policies Through Leadership, Collaboration, and Stakeholder Engagement

Nathan A. Shlobin, MD, MBA[a],*, Kemel A. Ghotme, MD, PhD[b,c],
Anastasia Arynchyna-Smith, MPH[d],*, Martina Gonzalez Gomez, MD[e],
Sarah Woodrow, MD[f], Jeffrey Blount, MD[e], Gail Rosseau, MD[g,h]

KEYWORDS

- Anencephaly • Folate fortification • Folic acid fortification • Global health • Global surgery
- Neural tube defects • Neurosurgical disease • Spina bifida

KEY POINTS

- Neurosurgical advocacy is an important avenue for facilitating legislation by translating research findings into concrete policy.
- The G4 Alliance and its member organizations have been involved in advocacy for folic acid fortification through the World Health Assembly since 2018.
- The G4 Alliance and its member organizations facilitated the adoption of a resolution to address micronutrient deficiencies through safe and effective food fortification to prevent congenital disorders such as spina bifida and anencephaly 76th World Health Assembly in 2023.

INTRODUCTION

Neural tube defects, primarily spina bifida and anencephaly (SBA), are common causes of mortality and morbidity among newborns. The global prevalence of spina bifida is 1 in 1000 births, while the prevalence of anencephaly is 1 in 4859 births worldwide,[1] with a higher prevalence in low- and middle-income countries (LMICs).[2] Level I evidence that has existed for over 30 years shows

[a] Department of Neurological Surgery, Northwestern University Feinberg School of Medicine, 710 West 168th Street, 4th Floor, New York, NY 10032, USA; [b] Translational Neuroscience Research Lab, Faculty of Medicine, Universidad de La Sabana, Carrera 7 No. 117 - 15, Bogota, Columbia; [c] Pediatric Neurosurgery, Department of Neurosurgery, Fundacion Santa Fe de Bogota, Campus del Puente del Común, Km. 7, Autopista Norte de Bogotá. Chía, Cundinamarca, Colombia; [d] Department of Neurosurgery, Division of Pediatric Neurosurgery, Children's of Alabama, University of Alabama at Birmingham, 1600 7th Avenue South, Lowder 400, Birmingham, AL 35233, USA; [e] Department of Neurosurgery, Division of Pediatric Neurosurgery, Children's of Alabama, University of Alabama at Birmingham, 1600 7th Avenue South, Lowder 400, Birmingham, AL 35233, USA; [f] Department of Neurological Surgery, Cleveland Clinic, Neuroscience Institute, 1 Akron General Avenue, Akron, OH 44307, USA; [g] Department of Neurological Surgery, George Washington University School of Medicine and Health Sciences, 2150 Pennsylvania Avenue, NW 7 South, Washington, DC 20037, USA; [h] Barrow Global, Barrow Neurological Institute, 2910 North Third Avenue, Phoenix, AZ 85013, USA
* Corresponding authors.
E-mail addresses: nshlobin@gmail.com (N.A.S.); arynch@uab.edu (A.A.-S.)
Twitter: @NathanShlobin (N.A.S.); @KemelG (K.A.G.); @Jpb1007Jeffrey (J.B.); @grosseaumd (G.R.)

Neurosurg Clin N Am 35 (2024) 411–420
https://doi.org/10.1016/j.nec.2024.05.003

that approximately 70% to 80% of SBA cases are preventable through adequate maternal folic acid (vitamin B9) consumption in the prenatal period.[3,4] Mandatory fortification with folic acid (FAF) is the most effective public health policy measure to ensure adequate folic acid intake. Variance in compliance, individual human behavior, and local/regional production of foods renders voluntary food fortification or folate supplementation consistently less effective.[5] However, only 61,680 folic acid-preventable cases of SBA were prevented in 2020 through mandatory FAF in 58 countries, representing only 22% of all preventable cases.[6] A large-scale approach is required to overcome the barriers and leverage the facilitating factors to implement this evidence-based policy.[7]

Neurosurgical advocacy constitutes an important avenue for facilitating policy initiatives, such as reducing inequities in preventable SBA.[8–10] The Global Alliance for Surgical, Obstetric, Trauma, and Anesthesia (SOTA) Care (G4 Alliance) and its member organizations have been heavily involved in neurosurgical advocacy, in part, through attending the annual World Health Assembly (WHA) since 2018.[11,12] In early 2022, the Global Alliance for the Prevention of Spina Bifida Folate (GAPSBiF), a member organization of the G4 Alliance, called for the urgent passage of a resolution at the WHA in favor of universal mandatory FAF.[13] The 75th WHA in 2022 saw expanding support for mandatory FAF as member organizations of the G4 Alliance presented a statement on its importance at the World Health Organization (WHO) 150th Executive Board Session.[14]

The G4 Alliance and its member organizations formed a neurosurgical delegation that participated in the 76th WHA (WHA76) in Geneva, Switzerland, in May 2023. This delegation facilitated the adoption of a new resolution focused on folic acid fortification to prevent SBA, the first neurosurgery-driven resolution since the founding of the WHO in 1948.[15] This landmark achievement required the coordination of stakeholders through global alliance for the prevention of spina bifida folate (GAPSBiF) and the G4 Alliance. In this study, we review and describe the role and landscape of neurosurgical advocacy, characterize advocacy for FAF to prevent SBA by highlighting the role of the G4 Alliance, and present future targets for advocacy initiatives to reduce SBA.

DISCUSSION
Neurosurgery in Global Health

Neurosurgical conditions result in substantial mortality and morbidity. Annually, 22.6 million patients experience neurologic disorders or injuries that require neurosurgical consultation, of whom 13.8 million require surgery.[16] The burden of neurosurgical disease is proportionately higher in LMICs.[17] An estimated 23,300 additional neurosurgeons are necessary to address unmet cases yearly in LMICs.[16] In locations like Sub-Saharan Africa, the number of neurosurgeons available to manage complex neurosurgical conditions is usually limited,[18] and other medical personnel are often similarly lacking. Barriers to delivering systems of neurosurgical care include inadequate funding, poor infrastructure, old or nonexistent equipment, lack of medicines, and deficiencies in the health system writ large. Moreover, challenges in accessing or affording neurosurgical care may prevent people from seeking neurosurgical care or force them to present at more advanced stages of the disease. Together, these factors result in more disability-adjusted life-years in LMICs.[17] Neurosurgical diseases are modeled to result in US$4.4 trillion in gross domestic product (GDP) losses during 2015 to 2030 in 90 LMICs.[19] Projected rapid population growth in LMICs over the next 30 years will likely exacerbate the incidence of congenital and pediatric diseases requiring neurosurgical care.[20] Population aging is also likely to increase the burden of neurosurgical disease in LMICs.[21] These factors will also likely increase necessary health care expenditures in LMICs.

If treated, neurosurgical conditions may reduce the global burden of disease, improve quality of life, and reduce extensive health care expenditures.[17,22] The Lancet Commission on Global Surgery launched the modern global surgery movement in 2015, which emphasized long-term solutions to the global burden of neurosurgical disease.[23] The WHA 68.15 resolution titled "Strengthening emergency and essential surgical care and anesthesia as a component of universal health coverage" further recognized the importance of global surgery as a discipline.[24] The Bogotá Declaration in 2016 heralded increased recognition that neurosurgeons worldwide must engage with policymakers to expand access to neurosurgical treatments.[18] The field of global neurosurgery represents the nexus of neurosurgery and public health and aims to reduce the global burden of neurosurgical disease through clinical practice, education, research, advocacy, and policy.[25] Since then, interest in global neurosurgery has grown rapidly.[26–28] The field has come to include students and trainees.[29,30]

As global neurosurgery has grown, there has been increased recognition that health systems-based efforts to address neurosurgical disease are necessary to ensure sustainable progress.[31] This represented a sharp divergence from the previous focus on short-term "mission-style" trips in international neurosurgery. Such short-term, stand-alone initiatives characteristically lacked follow-up and did not empower local health care personnel.[32] The realization that neurosurgical care pertains to 14 of the 17 United Nations (UN) Sustainable Development Goals (SDGs) announced in 2015 underpins this health systems approach.[33–35] Nonetheless, there are challenges. Health systems-focused literature in global neurosurgery remains lacking, with much of the current literature characterizing the global burden of neurosurgical disease.[31] Moreover, some collaborations between LMICs and high-income countries are inequitable.[28,36,37]

Neurosurgical Advocacy

Advocacy helps transform global health research into policy.[31] Advocacy occurs at the levels of international bodies and national, regional, and local governments.[30] There are a variety of stakeholders, including neurosurgeons, other physicians and health care personnel, policymakers, public health experts, and nongovernmental organizations.[30] Generation of political priority is a foundational aspect of neurosurgical advocacy.[38] A previous study has indicated that fragmentation, unifying leadership, an absence of guiding institutions, and disagreements regarding how to position global surgery have hampered global surgery efforts.[38] Insufficient mobilization of the momentum from the SDGs and public misconceptions regarding the cost and complexity of surgery have also contributed.[38] Neurosurgical advocacy must mitigate these factors to be successful.[30]

Advocacy in global neurosurgery has consisted of initiatives through neurosurgery-specific organizations or those that position global neurosurgery as a component of the wider global surgery or global health landscape.[30] The World Federation of Neurosurgical Societies (WFNS)–WHO Liaison Committee advocates for scaling up neurosurgical capacity globally at international meetings.[11,12] The G4 Alliance (https://www.theg4alliance.org/), a coalition of over 70 member organizations representing institutions, professional organizations, and nongovernmental organizations advocate broadly for increased access to safe and affordable surgical care. The G4 Alliance and other organizations do so by facilitating large-scale legislative action and supporting local initiatives, including national surgical, obstetric, and anesthesia planning, residency program establishment, and organization of surgical education.[39]

The WHO/WHA represents a pinnacle forum for large-scale neurosurgical advocacy.[11,12,14] Neurosurgical participation is essential as global health

care priorities are set and funding is organized at the WHA.[15] Resolutions indicate the WHO's commitment to a particular course of action but are nonbinding. After a resolution is discussed and accepted by the 34 WHO Executive Board (WHO-EB), the decision is presented to the WHA at large for discussion and approval.[15] Member states (MS) provide statements before the final decision to adopt or reject the resolution by the MS.[15] Written and oral statements on the floor of the WHA meeting highlight the relevance and importance of certain resolutions and the gravity of WHO-EB decisions.[15] Nonstate actors (NSA) who have official relations with the WHO may provide brief statements of support, opposition, or nuance but do not retain voting privileges.[15] In addition to the main WHA, various "side events" occur to develop new collaborations aimed at addressing key problems in global neurosurgery.[34,40]

Neurosurgical Advocacy for Food Fortification to Prevent Micronutrient Deficiencies

Since the founding of the modern global neurosurgery movement, evidence-based advocacy has been critical in areas such as helmet legislation, folate policy, and socioeconomic disparities.[5,17,41] FAF of staple foods represents, perhaps, the largest single advocacy issue in global neurosurgery. High-quality evidence exists regarding the efficacy of folate consumption in the prenatal and early pregnancy period,[3,4] as does evidence that mandatory FAF is the most effective way to ensure adequate folate consumption and can be easily tailored to the local diet.[5] However, the global lack of mandatory FAF policy implementation has led to an undue burden of SBA, especially in LMICs.[13] The avoidable mortality, morbidity, and health care expenditures on SBA compound the existing deficits in neurosurgical care in LMICs. A case study in Ethiopia indicated that FAF would prevent over 10,000 deaths associated with Spina Bifida (SB) and 10,000 stillbirths and save 37,800 surgical hours that could now be redirected to other neurosurgical cases, equivalent to 19 full-time equivalent neurosurgeon years.[42]

Neurosurgeons are well-equipped to advocate for preventing preventable neurosurgical conditions, such as SBA, and expanding safe, timely, and affordable neurosurgical care. Neurosurgeons are the primary caretakers of individuals with neurosurgical conditions and understand the trajectories of these neurosurgical diseases.[5] Their knowledge allows them to provide insight and recommendations regarding social, economic, and political factors that affect neurosurgical patients.[5] This is especially important in SBA care given the relevance of the context of the local diet, prenatal care, and FAF initiatives.[5] SBA represents the model condition for the dual approach of care provision and advocacy. Utilizing existing social and professional networks of neurosurgeon colleagues, other physicians, and public health personnel neurosurgical societies and organizations may foster a unique and united advocacy platform for public health initiatives.[5] The involvement of all stakeholders is essential to provide a comprehensive evidence base and complementary perspectives to advance the advocacy goals for FAF.

GAPSBiF (https://www.theg4alliance.org/gapsbif; https://sbf-forum.org/index.php) was founded in 2019 and accelerated its momentum in 2021. In 2021, the International Society for Pediatric Neurosurgery (ISPN) published a resolution advocating for mandatory FAF of staple foods to prevent SBA and associated disability and child mortality, with the goal of prevention of all preventable cases by 2030.[43] This resolution reflected the early experience in neurosurgeon-based advocacy of FAF in Costa Rica.[44–46] The Comprehensive Policy Recommendations for Spina Bifida and Hydrocephalus published by the Harvard Program in Global Surgery and Social Change together with ISPN has accelerated momentum for FAF.[47] GAPSBiF published an article in *The Lancet Global Health* calling for FAF to prevent SBA globally to garner wide readership across the global health community.[13]

At the 75th WHA, a statement titled "Global Prevention of Folic Acid-Preventable Spina Bifida and Anencephaly by 2030 by Prioritizing Food Fortification with Folic Acid" was introduced by the WFNS, World Federation of Societies of Anaesthesiologists, International Federation of Surgical Colleges, and International Federation of Gynecology and Obstetrics. The statement was approved at the 150th EB meeting.[15] The country of Colombia agreed to sponsor the proposed resolution. The 75th WHA also marked the approval of the WHO's Intersectoral Global Action Plan (IGAP) on Epilepsy and Other Neurological Disorders 2022-2031, guiding to prioritize the prevention and treatment of neurologic disorders,[48] echoing the commitments from the Bogotá Declaration.[15] Disease prevention, such as through FAF, constitutes an important objective of the IGAP.[48]

Folic Acid Fortification at the 76th World Health Assembly

WHA76 occurred in Geneva, Switzerland, in May 2023. The neurosurgical delegation consisted of 13 self-resourced neurosurgeons from Colombia, Costa Rica, Morocco, Pakistan, Spain, Turkey, and the United States who attended in person and many others who attended virtually.[15] The WHA76 represented the fourth year that a neurosurgery delegation joined the WHA, with many repeat attendees, deepening relationships between the neurosurgeons, WHO, ministers of health, and other global surgery partners.[15] The WFNS continued its position as an NSA with official relations with the WHO.[15] Neurosurgeons Dr Walter Johnson and Dr Kemel Ghotme functioned as WFNS delegates and submitted written and oral statements supporting 2 resolutions applicable to global surgery.[15] Dr Johnson previously led the Emergency and Essential Surgical Care Programme at the WHO from 2015 to 2019.

The first-ever neurosurgery-led resolution since the founding of the WHO in 1948 was developed and advanced by members of the GAPSBiF and the G4 Alliance.[15] Dr Kemel Ghotme, a Colombian pediatric neurosurgeon and translational medicine scholar, organized and led meetings with the Colombian Ministry of Health,[15] presenting them with key Level I evidence regarding the utility of FAF through the NeuroAdvocacy Toolkit.[49] After a comprehensive approach involving the Ministry of Health, Ministry of Foreign Affairs, and Permanent Mission in Geneva, Colombia decided to sponsor the resolution. The Colombian state representatives and the scientific community, represented by GAPSBiF, jointly devised a diplomatic route map to navigate the necessary steps to mobilize it to the WHA.[15] The resolution expanded from FAF to micronutrients following conversations with civil and government actors worldwide and consultation with technical experts at the WHO to provide increased reach and impact.[15] However, the resolution retained "spina bifida and other neural tube defects" in its title, given the neurosurgical relevance, visible neurologic disability, and multidisciplinary nature involving orthopedic, urologic, and gastrointestinal disabilities of these conditions.[15] Several rounds of edits on a draft resolution from October to December 2022 occurred. The Columbian diplomatic mission conducted science diplomacy activities with Dr Ghotme's scientific advice. The resolution entered the agenda for the WHO-EB meeting on February 3, 2023, as EB152/CONF./5, as part of the section on the UN Decade of Action on Nutrition.[15] In addition to initial sponsorship by Colombia, 37 other MS, including Australia, Brazil, Canada, Chile, Ecuador, the European Union, and its 27 MS, Israel, Malaysia, and Paraguay, provided cosponsorship.[15] The United States and Guatemala provided their support on the floor of the WHO-EB meeting.[15]

A letter signed by 80 multinational and neurosurgical organizations, academic institutions, scientific and professional organizations, and patient and family support networks highlighted broad public support for the resolution and was distributed to national delegates prior to the WHO-EB meeting.[15] The draft resolution was denoted as Decision EB152(13) and renamed "Accelerating efforts for preventing micronutrient deficiencies and their consequences, including spina bifida and other neural tube defects, through safe and effective food fortification." Colombia, Malaysia, and Ecuador partnered with GAPSBiF, the G4 Alliance, Global Alliance for Improved Nutrition (GAIN), International Federation for Spina Bifida and Hydrocephalus, Micronutrient Forum, Nutritional International, Reach Another Foundation, UN Children's Fund, and UN World Food Programme to conduct a campaign requesting that the 194 UN MS submit a written or oral floor statement in support of the resolution at WHA76.[15]

Additionally, the public-facing organizations cosponsored a side event at WHA76 focused on multidisciplinary support of the resolution.[15] WHO representatives, delegations from the Ministries of Health from Colombia, Malaysia, Ecuador, Ethiopia, Philippines, and Bangladesh, the neurosurgical community, the public health community, civil society, and—most importantly—people living with spina bifida participated.[15] The side event spurred further conversation and facilitated relationship-building between various stakeholders.[15] Moreover, the side event represented an additional aspect of the comprehensive, robust advocacy strategy aimed at securing support for the resolution to pass.[15]

On May 29, 2023, the WHA unanimously approved WHA76.19 (https://apps.who.int/gb/ebwha/pdf_files/WHA76/A76_R19-en.pdf), the micronutrient fortification resolution. Fifteen countries provided floor statements of support, and NSAs such as WFNS, GAIN, and others provided strong support as well.[50] Key events leading up to this approval are shown in **Fig. 1**.

Other World Health Assembly Resolutions Relevant to Neurosurgical Care

In addition to WHA76.19, the WHA adopted other resolutions relevant to neurosurgers. WHA76.2 ("Integrated emergency, critical and operative care [ECO] for universal health coverage and protection for health emergencies"), as cosponsored by 80 MS, highlighted that ECO services are foundational for strong health systems and the promotion of health equity.[51] WHA76.3 ("Increasing access to medical oxygen") emphasized the centrality of adequate oxygen supply to ensure safe surgical and anesthesia care.[52] WHA76.5 ("Strengthening the diagnostics

capacity") underscores the frequent absence of sufficient diagnostic equipment.[53] Neurosurgical diagnostic modalities such as computed tomography or MRI scanners are fundamental for modern practice. WHA 76.6 ("Strengthening rehabilitation in health systems") delineated the importance of rehabilitation in medical care.[54] Rehabilitation is a particularly important aspect of neurosurgery given the impacts of neurologic disease on cognitive functioning, speech, activities of daily living, and mobility.

Altogether, the WHA resolutions relevant to neurosurgery provided key takeaways. First, the role of neurosurgical care in global health is not limited to its operative components. Undoubtedly, neurosurgical conditions require timely and adequate operative care. However, the entire patient pathway is essential, from diagnosis to rehabilitation. Initiatives solely focused on the operative aspect of neurosurgery are likely to provide limited and unsustainable impact.

Second, neurosurgery is part of the wider unified global health and surgery fronts. Most neurosurgical diseases are quite disabling and require multidisciplinary care. Congenital disorders lead to particularly long-term effects on health, psychosocial outcomes, and health care expenditures. For example, care for patients with SB involves the expertise of orthopedic surgeons, urologists, gastroenterologists, general surgeons, and physical therapists.[55–57] Collective advocacy by multidisciplinary stakeholders, which may be neurosurgeon-led, as with GAPSBiF, may be the most effective structure for advancing policy objectives. These stakeholders include other physicians and health care personnel, subject matter experts, professional and patient support societies, local personnel, and civil society.[15] Neurosurgeon-only advocacy will likely contribute to already fragmented advocacy initiatives and miss the valuable perspectives of other individuals caring for people with neurosurgical conditions. Advocacy should occur at the international and national levels in addition to at the local level. Moreover, given there are relatively few neurosurgeons, collaborating with other physicians and personnel will allow neurosurgeons to achieve a common goal, such as advancing health equity. Neurosurgeons will have a stronger, more unified voice, as well as greater political power.

Third, safe, timely, and affordable neurosurgical care is essential to strengthening health systems. Neurosurgical conditions are responsible for much of the overall global burden of disease and ensuing health care expenditures.[16,19,58] Brain tumors, spinal tumors, hydrocephalus, and neural tube defects warrant neurosurgical consultation and operative intervention with high frequency.[59]

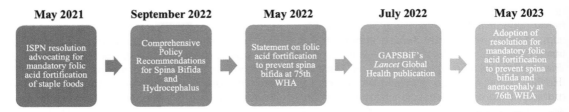

Fig. 1. Key events leading up to adoption of folic acid fortification at the WHA76. GAPSBiF, Global Alliance for Prevention of Spina Bifida Folate; ISPN, International Society for Pediatric Neurosurgery; WHA, World Health Assembly.

Health systems must be equipped with strong neurosurgical care infrastructure at the acute, subacute, and chronic periods and sufficient neurosurgeons and other health care personnel to address these neurosurgical conditions adequately. Neurosurgeons must advocate for initiatives that strengthen health systems in addition to neurosurgery-specific topics.

Other Events at the 76th World Health Assembly Attended by the Neurosurgical Delegation

The theme for WHA76 was "WHO at 75: Saving lives, driving health for all." WHA76 opened with the annual Walk the Talk event to affirm solidarity for the WHO's goals while keeping participants active.[15] WHO Director-General Dr Tedros Adhanom Ghebreyesus began the event with a speech on the importance of serving as champions for universal health coverage.[15] The neurosurgical delegation discussed the progress of the WHO related to surgical care with Dr Tedros and health ministers from participant countries.[15]

The G4 Alliance has served as the "home" for neurosurgery and SOTA groups during the WHA.[15] The G4 Alliance held its 13th meeting of the Permanent Council and working group meetings immediately preceding the WHA.[15] The Permanent Council defined 4 primary calls to action for MS of the WHO and the international community, including (1) SOTA care for all in the postpandemic time, (2) multidisciplinary collaboration in SOTA care, (3) responding to growing health care shortages due to brain drain and weak infrastructure coupled with an expanding yet aging population, and (4) the intersection of SOTA care with primary health care and its role in universal health coverage.[15]

The G4 Alliance organized 2 side events focused on policy pathways to improve surgical care access, quality, and affordability.[15] First, the G4 Alliance member organizations and the Southern African Development Community Technical Experts Working Group on Surgical Healthcare cohosted "Resolutions to Reality: Bringing Surgery & Anaesthesia into Primary Health Care," which characterized the benefit of incorporating surgical care into national and subnational primary health care approaches.[15] Government representatives from Ethiopia and Peru, WHO staff, the Laerdal Foundation, and hosting organization members participated in the panel.[15] Second, the G4 Alliance and the Accreditation Council for Graduate Medical Education International cohosted "Suturing the Gaps in Global Workforce for Surgical Care" to shed light on strengthening the workforce of surgeons, other physicians, and other health care personnel and staff and the fundamental nature of a patient-centered approach to surgical care.[15] Additionally, individual member organizations of the G4 Alliance held events. As mentioned, GAPSBiF held a session on the WHA micronutrient fortification resolution.[15] InterSurgeon (www.intersurgeon.org), a virtual platform that seeks to connect individuals and organizations involved in global surgery,[60] organized a session emphasizing the platform's utility for G4 Alliance member organizations in expanding their operations and facilitating SOTA care.[15] Operation Smile (https://www.operationsmile.org/), a global nonprofit organization devoted to safe surgery, comprehensive medical care for people with cleft lip and palate, and strong advocacy for SOTA care for all, celebrated its 40th anniversary with a side event.[15] This event emphasized the utility of partnerships in global surgery, the transformative role of women in medicine and global health, and Operation Smile's vision for its next decade.[15]

The Global Surgery Foundation hosted a side event panel regarding the urgent need for financial resources to scale up surgical systems capacity.[15] Dr Phumzile Mlambo-Ngcuka, the former Deputy President of South Africa and Executive Director of UN Women, highlighted the urgent importance of increasing access to surgical care among women.[15] Dr Rifat Atun of the Harvard T.H. Chan School of Public Health announced the SURGfund (https://www.globalsurgeryfoundation.org/surgfund), the Global Surgery Foundation's catalytic funding mechanism.[15] Dr Atul Gawande characterized the United States Agency for International Development's progress over the previous year and its plans for the year 2023 to 2024.[15] Ms Nácia Pupo Taylor, the Senior Director of Global Public Health at Johnson & Johnson, committed to supporting SurgHub (www.surghub.org), the UN Global Surgery Learning Hub.[15]

Future Directions for Neurosurgical Advocacy

A unique opportunity exists for neurosurgeons to advocate for the prevention of neurosurgical conditions and access to neurosurgical care. Future advocacy initiatives should retain their multidisciplinary approach. The WHA76.19 resolution highlights the potential success of such a multidisciplinary approach.[50,52,61] However, a resolution alone is insufficient. Nonbinding resolutions do not entail concrete action and are often ineffective due to a lack of follow-up. Neurosurgeons must utilize WHA76.19 to motivate action in their countries and regions toward mandatory FAF. Highlighting the view of experts on the efficacy of FAF and supporting the global health community of FAF while addressing local social, political, economic, cultural, and linguistic factors will be useful. As the unified representation of all 194 MS, the WHO must provide logistical, technical, and material support to facilitate policy implementation, surveillance, and long-term sustainability.[15] In general, the WHA76.19 stands out as an example of the importance of neurosurgical advocacy to motivate future advocacy efforts in areas such as helmet legislation, violence, and strengthening health systems.

SUMMARY

The passage of the resolution on micronutrient fortification of staple foods to prevent SBA and other NTDs at the WHA76 represents a landmark in neurosurgical advocacy as the first neurosurgeon-led resolution at the WHA. Coupled with other resolutions and side events relevant to neurosurgery, this resolution cements a commitment to FAF to prevent SBA to reduce morbidity, mortality, and health care expenditures and broadens the focus on neurosurgery as an important component of global surgery. Neurosurgeons must leverage this opportunity as critical constituents of multidisciplinary teams to generate policy aimed at preventing neurosurgical diseases and injuries, and ensuring access to safe, timely, and affordable neurosurgical care to all people.

ACKNOWLEDGMENTS

This article is written on behalf of the Global Alliance for the Prevention of Spina Bifida Folate (GAPSBiF). The authors acknowledge Roxanna Garcia, MD, MS, MPH; Walter D. Johnson, MD; Frederick A. Boop, MD; Kee B. Park, MD, MPH; Adrian Caceres, MD; Rosa A. Pardo Vargas, MD; Ruben Ayala, MD, MSc; Geoffrey Ibbotson, MD; Natalie Sheneman, BA; Daniel B. Peterson, MBA; Eylen Öcal, MD; Arsene Daniel Nyalunja, MD; Jesus La Fuente, MD; Tariq Khan, MD; Laura J. Hobart-Porter, DO; Richard P. Moser, MD; Yakob S. Ahmed, MPH, MBA; Najia El Abbadi, MD, PhD; Kristin Sundell, MDiv; Saskia J.M. Osendarp, PhD, MSc; Homero Martinez, PhD for their work at the WHA76 and contribution to a recent article foundational to the present article, "Global Neurosurgery at the 76th World Health Assembly (2023): First Neurosurgery-Driven Resolution Calls for Micronutrient Fortification to Prevent Spina Bifida."

DISCLOSURE

The authors have nothing to disclose.

REFERENCES

1. Blencowe H, Kancherla V, Moorthie S, et al. Estimates of global and regional prevalence of neural tube defects for 2015: a systematic analysis. Ann N Y Acad Sci 2018;1414(1):31–46.
2. Lo A, Polšek D, Sidhu S. Estimating the burden of neural tube defects in low–and middle–income countries. Journal of Global health 2014;4(1).
3. Group MVSR. Prevention of neural tube defects: results of the Medical Research Council Vitamin Study. Lancet 1991;338(8760):131–7.
4. Czeizel AE, Dudas I. Prevention of the first occurrence of neural-tube defects by periconceptional vitamin supplementation. N Engl J Med 1992;327(26):1832–5.
5. Shlobin NA, LoPresti MA, Du RY, et al. Folate fortification and supplementation in prevention of folate-sensitive neural tube defects: a systematic review of policy. J Neurosurg Pediatr 2020;27(3):294–310.
6. Kancherla V, Wagh K, Priyadarshini P, et al. A global update on the status of prevention of folic acid-preventable spina bifida and anencephaly in year 2020: 30-Year anniversary of gaining knowledge about folic acid's prevention potential for neural tube defects. Birth Defects Research 2022;114(20):1392–403.
7. Ghotme KA, Arynchyna-Smith A, Maleknia P, et al. Barriers and facilitators to the implementation of mandatory folate fortification as an evidence-based policy to prevent neural tube defects. Child's Nerv Syst 2023;1–8.

8. Estevez-Ordonez D, Davis MC, Hopson B, et al. Reducing inequities in preventable neural tube defects: the critical and underutilized role of neurosurgical advocacy for folate fortification. Neurosurg Focus 2018;45(4):E20.

9. Shlobin NA, Roach JT, Kancherla V, et al. The role of neurosurgeons in global public health: the case of folic acid fortification of staple foods to prevent spina bifida. J Neurosurg Pediatr 2022;1(aop):1–8.

10. Shlobin NA, Ghotme K, Caceres A, et al. Neurosurgeon-Led Advocacy for Folic Acid Fortification to Prevent Spina Bifida. World Neurosurgery 2023; 172:96–7.

11. Rosseau G, Johnson WD, Park KB, et al. Global neurosurgery: current and potential impact of neurosurgeons at the World Health Organization and the World Health Assembly. Executive summary of the World Federation of Neurosurgical Societies–World Health Organization Liaison Committee at the 71st World Health Assembly. Neurosurg Focus 2018; 45(4):E18.

12. Rosseau G, Johnson WD, Park KB, et al. Global neurosurgery: continued momentum at the 72nd World Health Assembly. J Neurosurg 2020;132(4): 1256–60.

13. Kancherla V, Botto LD, Rowe LA, et al. Preventing birth defects, saving lives, and promoting health equity: an urgent call to action for universal mandatory food fortification with folic acid. Lancet Glob Health 2022;10(7):e1053–7.

14. Garcia RM, Ghotme KA, Arynchyna-Smith A, et al. Global Neurosurgery: Progress and Resolutions at the 75th World Health Assembly. Neurosurgery 2022;10:1227.

15. Gomez MG, Arynchyna-Smith A, Ghotme KA, et al. Global Neurosurgery at the 76th World Health Assembly (2023): First Neurosurgery-driven Resolution Calls for Micronutrient Fortification to Prevent Spina Bifida. World Neurosurgery 2024;185:135–40.

16. Dewan MC, Rattani A, Fieggen G, et al. Global neurosurgery: the current capacity and deficit in the provision of essential neurosurgical care. Executive Summary of the Global Neurosurgery Initiative at the Program in Global Surgery and Social Change. J Neurosurg 2018;130(4):1055–64.

17. Veerappan VR, Gabriel PJ, Shlobin NA, et al. Global Neurosurgery in the Context of Global Public Health Practice–A Literature Review of Case Studies. World Neurosurgery 2022;165:20–6.

18. Punchak M, Mukhopadhyay S, Sachdev S, et al. Neurosurgical Care: Availability and Access in Low-Income and Middle-Income Countries. World Neurosurg 2018;112:e240–54.

19. Rudolfson N, Dewan MC, Park KB, et al. The economic consequences of neurosurgical disease in low-and middle-income countries. J Neurosurg 2018;130(4):1149–56.

20. Nations U. Global issues: Population. Available at: https://www.un.org/en/global-issues/population. [Accessed 7 June 2023].

21. Gyasi RM, Phillips DR. Aging and the rising burden of noncommunicable diseases in sub-Saharan Africa and other low-and middle-income countries: a call for holistic action. Gerontol 2020;60(5):806–11.

22. Rubiano AM, Vera DS, Montenegro JH, et al. Recommendations of the Colombian Consensus Committee for the Management of Traumatic Brain Injury in Prehospital, Emergency Department, Surgery, and Intensive Care (Beyond One Option for Treatment of Traumatic Brain Injury: A Stratified Protocol [BOOTStraP]). J Neurosci Rural Pract 2020; 11(1):7–22.

23. Meara JG, Leather AJ, Hagander L, et al. Global Surgery 2030: evidence and solutions for achieving health, welfare, and economic development. Lancet 2015;386(9993):569–624.

24. Organization WH. Strengthening emergency and essential surgical care and anaesthesia as a component of universal health coverage. 2015. Available at: https://apps.who.int/gb/ebwha/pdf_files/WHA68/A68 _R15-en.pdf. [Accessed 10 July 2023].

25. Park KB, Johnson WD, Dempsey RJ. Global Neurosurgery: The Unmet Need. World Neurosurg 2016; 88:32–5.

26. Hansen RTB, Hansen RAB, Behmer VA, et al. Update on the global neurosurgery movement: a systematic review of international vernacular, research trends, and authorship. J Clin Neurosci 2020;79:183–90.

27. Niquen-Jimenez M, Wishart D, Garcia RM, et al. A bibliographic analysis of the most cited articles in global neurosurgery. World neurosurgery 2020; 144:e195–203.

28. Paradie E, Warman PI, Waguia-Kouam R, et al. The scope, growth, and inequities of the global neurosurgery literature: a bibliometric analysis. World Neurosurgery 2022;167:e670–84.

29. Zolo Y, de Koning R, Ozair A, et al. Medical students in global neurosurgery: rationale and role. Journal of Global Neurosurgery 2021;1(1):25–9.

30. Shlobin NA, Kanmounye US, Ozair A, et al. Educating the next generation of global neurosurgeons: competencies, skills, and resources for medical students interested in global neurosurgery. World neurosurgery 2021;155:150–9.

31. Ham EI, Kim J, Kanmounye US, et al. Cohesion between research literature and health system level efforts to address global neurosurgical inequity: a scoping review. World Neurosurgery 2020;143: e88–105.

32. Dempsey RJ, Buckley NA. Education-based solutions to the global burden of neurosurgical disease. World neurosurgery 2020;140:e1–6.

33. Nations U. Sustainable Development Goals. 2023. Available at: https://www.un.org/sustainabledevelop

ment/development-agenda/#:~:text=The%2017%20Goals%20were%20adopted,the%20speed%20or%20scale%20required. [Accessed 31 July 2023].

34. Lartigue JW, Dada OE, Haq M, et al. Emphasizing the Role of Neurosurgery Within Global Health and National Health Systems: A Call to Action. Front Surg 2021;8:690735.

35. Barthélemy EJ, Park KB, Johnson W. Neurosurgery and Sustainable Development Goals. World Neurosurg 2018;120:143–52.

36. Ukachukwu A-EK, Seas A, Petitt Z, et al. Assessing the Success and Sustainability of Global Neurosurgery Collaborations: Systematic Review and Adaptation of the Framework for Assessment of InteRNational Surgical Success Criteria. World Neurosurgery 2022;167:111–21.

37. Cannizzaro D, Safa A, Bisoglio A, et al. Second Footprint of Reports from Low-and Low-to Middle-Income Countries in the Neurosurgical Data: A Study from 2018–2020 Compared with Data from 2015–2017. World Neurosurgery 2022;168: e666–74.

38. Shawar YR, Shiffman J, Spiegel DA. Generation of political priority for global surgery: a qualitative policy analysis. Lancet Global Health 2015;3(8): e487–95.

39. Kanmounye US, Shenaman N, Ratel M, et al. A seat at the table: representation of global neurosurgery in the G4 alliance. Journal of Global Neurosurgery 2021;1(1):73–7.

40. Uche EO, Sundblom J, Uko UK, et al. Global neurosurgery over a 60-year period: Conceptual foundations, time reference, emerging Co-ordinates and prospects for collaborative interventions in low and middle income countries. Brain Spine 2022;2:101187.

41. Du RY, LoPresti MA, García RM, et al. Primary prevention of road traffic accident–related traumatic brain injuries in younger populations: a systematic review of helmet legislation. J Neurosurg Pediatr 2020;25(4):361–74.

42. Kancherla V, Koning J, Biluts H, et al. Projected impact of mandatory food fortification with folic acid on neurosurgical capacity needed for treating spina bifida in Ethiopia. Birth defects research 2021;113(5):393–8.

43. Caceres A, Blount JP, Messing-Jünger M, et al. The International Society for Pediatric Neurosurgery resolution on mandatory folic acid fortification of staple foods for prevention of spina bifida and anencephaly and associated disability and child mortality. Childs Nerv Syst 2021;37(6):1809–12.

44. Caceres A, Jimenez-Chaverri AL, Alpizar-Quiros PA, et al. Pre and postnatal care characteristics and management features of children born with myelomeningocele in the post-folate fortification era of staple foods in Costa Rica (2004-2022). Childs Nerv Syst 2023;39(7):1755–64.

45. Caceres A, Blount JP. Preventing spina bifida through folate fortification: a labor of love. Childs Nerv Syst 2023;39(7):1695–7.

46. Benavides-Lara A, Fernández-Sánchez O, Barboza-Argüello MP, et al. Integrated surveillance strategy to support the prevention of neural tube defects through food fortification with folic acid: the experience of Costa Rica. Childs Nerv Syst 2023;39(7): 1743–54.

47. Pattisapu JV, Veerappan VR, White C, et al. Spina bifida management in low-and middle-income countries—a comprehensive policy approach. Child's Nerv Syst 2023;1–9.

48. Gupta S, Aukrust CG, Bhebhe A, et al. Neurosurgery and the World Health Organization Intersectoral Global Action Plan for Epilepsy and Other Neurological Disorders 2022–2031. Neurosurgery 2022;10: 1227.

49. Ghotme KA. The NeuroAdvocacy Toolkit: a knowledge translation strategy to strengthen food fortification Policies to prevent neural tube defects in Latin American countries. A mixed-method study. Washington, DC: Washington University; 2023. Available at: https://hsrc.himmelfarb.gwu.edu/smhs_crl_dissertations/18/.

50. Organization WH. Accelerating efforts for preventing micronutrient deficiencies and their consequences, including spina bifida and other neural tube defects, through safe and effective food fortification. 2023. Available at: https://apps.who.int/gb/ebwha/pdf_files/WHA76/A76_R19-en.pdf. [Accessed 21 June 2023].

51. Organization WH. Surgical and Anaesthesia Care. 2023. Available at: https://www.who.int/teams/integrated-health-services/clinical-services-and-systems/surgical-care. [Accessed 21 June 2023].

52. Organization WH. Increasing access to medical oxygen. 2023. Available at: https://apps.who.int/gb/ebwha/pdf_files/WHA76/A76_R3-en.pdf. [Accessed 21 June 2023].

53. Organization WH. Strengthening diagnostics capacity. 2023. Available at: https://apps.who.int/gb/ebwha/pdf_files/WHA76/A76_R5-en.pdf. [Accessed 21 June 2023].

54. Organization WH. Strengthening rehabilitation in health systems. 2023. Available at: https://apps.who.int/gb/ebwha/pdf_files/WHA76/A76_R6-en.pdf. [Accessed 21 June 2023].

55. Alabi NB, Thibadeau J, Wiener JS, et al. Surgeries and health outcomes among patients with spina bifida. Pediatrics 2018;142(3):e20173730.

56. Shlobin NA, Yerkes EB, Swaroop VT, et al. Multidisciplinary spina bifida clinic: the Chicago experience. Child's Nerv Syst 2022;38(9):1675–81.

57. Reynolds RA, Vance EH, Shlobin NA, et al. Transitioning care for adolescents with spina bifida in the US: challenges for management. Child's Nerv Syst 2023;1–8.

58. O'Donohoe T, Choudhury A, Callander E. Global macroeconomic burden of epilepsy and the role for neurosurgery: a modelling study based upon the 2016 Global Burden of Disease data. Eur J Neurol 2020;27(2):360–8.

59. Dewan MC, Rattani A, Baticulon RE, et al. Operative and consultative proportions of neurosurgical disease worldwide: estimation from the surgeon perspective. J Neurosurg 2018;130(4): 1098–106.

60. Maleknia P, Shlobin NA, Johnston Jr JM, et al. Establishing collaborations in global neurosurgery: The role of InterSurgeon. J Clin Neurosci 2022;100: 164–8.

61. Organization WH. Integrated emergency, critical and operative care for universal health coverage and protection from health emergencies. 2023. Available at: https://apps.who.int/gb/ebwha/pdf_files/WHA76/A76_R2-en.pdf. [Accessed 21 June 2023].

Partnering in Global Health
What Is a Successful Dyad? The Duke Experience

Anthony T. Fuller, MD, MScGH[a,b,1],
Michael M. Haglund, MD, PhD, MEd, MACM[a,c,d],*

KEYWORDS

- Global neurosurgery • Dyad • Duke global neurosurgery and neurology • Uganda
- Capacity building • Training and education • Research and innovation • Sustainable partnerships

KEY POINTS

- The Duke Global Neurosurgery and Neurology-Uganda dyad highlights the critical role of international collaborations in enhancing global neurosurgical care.
- Significant accomplishments include the establishment of a neurosurgery residency program, expansion of neurosurgical services, and the development of an epilepsy clinic.
- Overcoming challenges such as resource constraints and navigating cross-cultural collaborations were pivotal to the dyad's success.
- Sustainable impact in global neurosurgery requires a focus on service, training, research, and developing self-sustaining health care models.

INTRODUCTION

In the vast and interconnected world of health care, the essence of partnership stands as a beacon of hope, illuminating the path toward a more equitable and accessible global neurosurgery landscape. It is here, within the framework of collaborative engagement, that we find the power of global neurosurgery dyads—partnerships meticulously formed between entities striving for a shared vision of improving neurosurgical care in regions where the need is most acute. The question is not why we should embark on such partnerships but, rather, how we can afford not to. In the spirit of unity and shared purpose, these partnerships offer a blueprint for overcoming inequities.

The call for collaboration in global neurosurgery has never been more urgent.[1–5] As we navigate the complexities of delivering high-quality health care across increasingly porous borders, the importance of strategic partnerships, particularly in neurosurgery, becomes increasingly clear. These alliances, especially those formed between academic institutions and health care providers in low-income and middle-income countries, are not merely beneficial; they are essential. They serve as a conduit for sharing knowledge, resources, and innovations, amplifying our ability to address the dire need for surgical services worldwide.[6,7] The concept of a dyad, a partnership between 2 entities, emerges as a powerful strategy for making tangible progress in this endeavor.[8,9] By pooling expertise and resources, dyads can achieve outcomes that would be unattainable by either party acting alone.

[a] Duke Global Neurosurgery and Neurology, Durham, NC, USA; [b] Fuller Health Solutions, Salt Lake City, UT, USA; [c] Duke University Global Health Institute, Durham, NC, USA; [d] Department of Neurosurgery, Duke Health, 4508 Hospital South, Durham, NC 27710, USA
[1] Present address: 250 East 200 South, Salt Lake City, UT 84111.
* Corresponding author.
E-mail address: michael.haglund@duke.edu

Neurosurg Clin N Am 35 (2024) 421–428
https://doi.org/10.1016/j.nec.2024.05.004
1042-3680/24/© 2024 Elsevier Inc. All rights are reserved, including those for text and data mining, AI training, and similar technologies.

Furthermore, establishing such partnerships goes beyond the immediate benefits of enhanced neurosurgical care. They embody a deeper commitment to equity, capacity building, and the sharing of best practices across the globe. In regions where neurosurgical services are scarce or nonexistent, the impact of these partnerships can be life-changing for the patients who receive care and for local health care professionals who gain invaluable skills and knowledge.[10,11] This exchange fosters an environment of mutual learning and respect, where innovations in neurosurgery can flourish and adapt to meet the unique needs of diverse populations.

At the heart of these endeavors is a shared vision of a world where access to quality neurosurgical care is a reality for everyone, regardless of geographic location or socioeconomic status.[12] This vision compels us to consider the role of partnerships not as optional but as fundamental to advancing global neurosurgery. In this article, the authors reflect on the successes, challenges, and lessons learned through the dyadic partnership between Duke Global Neurosurgery and Neurology (DGNN) and Uganda. The authors share their experience to offer a roadmap and guide for navigating partnerships in global neurosurgery. The authors hope their experience reminds readers that in the vast and interconnected world of health care, our greatest strength lies in our ability to come together, share our knowledge, and work toward a common purpose.

THE DUKE GLOBAL NEUROSURGERY AND NEUROLOGY-UGANDA DYAD
The Genesis of Partnership

The journey of the DGNN and Uganda partnership began not as a mere coincidence but as a deliberate and thoughtful union of shared objectives and mutual respect. It was born out of a recognition that combining both entities' expertise, resources, and passion could transform the dream of enhancing neurosurgical care in Uganda into reality.

The genesis of the DGNN and Uganda partnership is a testament to the power of intentional collaboration and shared vision. This alliance resulted from deliberate efforts on both sides with a shared understanding of Uganda's critical need for enhanced neurosurgical capabilities.[10,13] Recognizing the disparities in neurosurgical care between different parts of the world,[14–16] there was an opportunity to make a significant impact by pooling resources, knowledge, and passion for health care improvement. The partnership was built on mutual respect, with both parties committed to listening, learning, and adapting to each other's needs and perspectives. This approach ensured that the collaboration was not only about transferring knowledge and resources from Duke to Uganda but also about creating a reciprocal relationship where both parties could grow and learn from the experience.

The initial conversations and meetings were characterized by a deep sense of optimism and a shared belief in the potential of what could be achieved together. Early discussions focused on understanding the challenges faced by the Ugandan health care system, particularly in neurosurgery, and how the DGNN could best support and enhance the existing infrastructure and training programs. This partnership phase involved a lot of listening, with DGNN team members spending time in Uganda to gain a firsthand understanding of the local context and needs.[17–22] It was during these early days that the partnership's goals were crystallized—to improve the availability and quality of neurosurgical care in Uganda through capacity building, training, and research.[21] The commitment to these goals, grounded in a spirit of partnership and mutual respect, laid the foundation for the transformative work that would follow.

The Focus of the Partnership

The partnership between DGNN and Uganda began using the "4 T's paradigm," which consisted of technology, twinning, training, and a top-down approach.[21] The partnership has since refocused its approach and has strategically concentrated its efforts across 3 pivotal areas: service, research, and training.[13] This multifaceted approach ensures a comprehensive and sustainable impact on Uganda's neurosurgical landscape. Service initiatives featuring neurosurgical camps that provide much-needed surgical interventions in underserved areas have been a cornerstone of the partnership.[10] Additionally, the partnership has facilitated the donation of critical neurosurgical equipment and supplies, significantly enhancing the capacity of local health care facilities to deliver high-quality neurosurgical care.

Research has played a crucial role in understanding and addressing the unique challenges of neurosurgery in Uganda. The partnership has embarked on a wide array of research projects, covering topics from the epidemiology of neurologic disorders within the region to in-hospital outcomes and the effectiveness of community-based care.[11,23] This research is not only aimed at gathering insights but also at informing practices and policies that can improve neurosurgical care outcomes.[24–27] By focusing on evidence-based interventions and outcomes, the partnership ensures that its efforts are guided by data and best practices, contributing to the global body of knowledge in neurosurgery.

Training is another critical component of the partnership's focus, recognizing that building local capacity is essential for long-term sustainability. A major achievement in this area has been developing a neurosurgery residency program designed to cultivate the next generation of neurosurgeons in Uganda.[10,28,29] Additionally, the partnership has invested in the training of biomedical technicians, crucial for the maintenance of neurosurgical equipment, and in the training of health care professionals in epilepsy management.[30–32] This comprehensive training approach ensures that all cadres of staff involved in neurosurgery care, from surgeons to nurses and technicians, are equipped with the knowledge and skills to provide exceptional care.

By addressing these 3 areas—service, research, and training—the DGNN and Uganda partnership is creating a robust foundation for advancing neurosurgical care in Uganda. Through neurosurgical camps and equipment donations, the partnership directly enhances service delivery. Through targeted research initiatives, it contributes to a deeper understanding of the challenges and solutions in neurosurgery. And through extensive training programs it builds the local capacity necessary for sustainable health improvements. Together, these efforts mark a significant stride toward ensuring that quality neurosurgical care is accessible to all those in need within the region, ultimately aiming to transform the right to neurosurgical care from a privilege into a reality for the people of Uganda.

Major Accomplishments

The partnership between DGNN and Uganda has achieved remarkable successes that have significantly impacted the neurosurgical landscape in Uganda and beyond. Among the most profound accomplishments is the number of patient lives saved and improved through direct interventions and enhanced care capabilities. Through neurosurgical camps, improved local facilities, and the introduction of advanced surgical techniques, countless individuals have received life-saving treatments for previously untreated conditions.[22] This direct impact on patient lives underscores the partnership's primary mission: to make neurosurgical care accessible and effective for all who need it.

Another cornerstone achievement of the partnership is the establishment of a neurosurgery residency program in Uganda. This program is pivotal in addressing the critical shortage of neurosurgeons in the region.[29,33–35] By training local health care professionals within their community, the program ensures the sustainability of neurosurgical care in Uganda, empowering local professionals to lead and further develop the field. The residency program has not only increased the number of qualified neurosurgeons in the area but also fostered a culture of continuous learning and improvement within the local health care system. There are now enough neurosurgeons in Uganda that they have developed a neurosurgical society—The Neurosurgical Society of Uganda.

Expanding neurosurgery services across Uganda marks another significant milestone for the partnership. Before this collaboration, neurosurgical services were limited and concentrated in a few locations.[21] Now, thanks to the efforts of the DGNN and Uganda partnership, multiple locations across the country can offer specialized neurosurgical services. This expansion has dramatically increased access to care for patients, reducing the need for long and often prohibitive travel to receive treatment. Furthermore, establishing an epilepsy clinic has provided focused care for patients with epilepsy, offering diagnosis, management, and ongoing support tailored to their specific needs.[36–38] This clinic has become a model for comprehensive care that could be replicated in other regions.

The partnership's commitment to education and research has also yielded significant accomplishments. The partnership has profoundly increased the capacity for neurosurgical care in Uganda by training various health care professionals, including surgeons, nurses, technicians, and community health workers. The breadth and depth of research outputs generated by this collaboration are impressive, encompassing abstracts, posters, conference presentations, manuscripts, book chapters, and special issues of journals. These contributions have not only advanced the global understanding of neurosurgery but also positioned the DGNN and Uganda partnership as leaders in neurosurgical research and education.[5] Through these achievements, the partnership demonstrates the power of collaboration, innovation, and dedication in transforming the landscape of global neurosurgery.

Financing the Partnership

Financing the partnership has been a critical component of its success. The partnership has utilized a diverse portfolio of funding sources, including grants from governmental and nongovernmental organizations, philanthropic donations from individuals and foundations, and institutional support from Duke University and other institutions. This multifaceted approach to funding has enabled the partnership to undertake ambitious projects in service, research, and training, ensuring that its initiatives are well-supported and sustainable over the long term.

Grants have played a pivotal role in supporting the partnership's research endeavors, allowing for the exploration of key issues in neurosurgery and the development of innovative solutions to improve patient outcomes. These grants, awarded by bodies dedicated to advancing medical research and global health, have facilitated studies ranging from epidemiology to the effectiveness of specific neurosurgical interventions. Such research is essential for enhancing the quality of care within Uganda and contributing valuable insights to the global medical community.

Philanthropic donations have been instrumental in expanding the service and training aspects of the partnership. Generous contributions from individuals and foundations have funded neurosurgical camps, provided critical medical supplies and equipment, and supported the development of training programs for Ugandan health care professionals. This philanthropic support reflects a broad-based commitment to improving global health outcomes. It underscores the vital role that individual and collective generosity plays in advancing medical care in underserved areas.

Institutional support from Duke University and other institutions has provided a solid foundation for the partnership's ongoing operations and future initiatives. This support includes not only financial backing but also the provision of expertise, facilities, and logistical assistance. The commitment of these institutions to the partnership's mission has been crucial in building and maintaining the infrastructure necessary for its success, from training centers to clinical facilities.

DISCUSSION
Challenges Overcome

The journey of the DGNN and Uganda partnership has navigated a landscape rife with challenges, each presenting unique hurdles to the mission of enhancing neurosurgical care. Resource constraints initially posed a significant barrier, with limited access to medical supplies, equipment, and financial support hampering the ability to deliver care and conduct training. Moreover, the complexities of cross-cultural collaboration required careful negotiation and understanding, as both teams from Duke and Uganda worked to align their approaches, expectations, and methodologies in health care delivery and education. Despite these obstacles, the partnership has leveraged resilience and adaptability, turning potential setbacks into opportunities for growth and innovation.

In overcoming these hurdles, the partnership has exemplified the power of collective resolve and the importance of a flexible approach to problem-solving. Strategies such as engaging local stakeholders, sourcing alternative funding, and utilizing technology for training and communication have been instrumental in mitigating resource limitations. Additionally, the emphasis on cultural exchange and mutual learning has enriched the collaboration, allowing both parties to gain deeper insights into each other's working environments and health care systems. This mutual understanding has been pivotal in crafting interventions and training programs that are effective and, culturally and contextually, relevant.

The success in overcoming these challenges has not only advanced the partnership's objectives but also served as a beacon of inspiration for similar initiatives globally. The DGNN and Uganda partnership underscores the importance of perseverance, adaptability, and a commitment to shared goals by demonstrating that obstacles can be transformed into catalysts for innovation and deeper collaboration. These lessons highlight the essential components of successful international health care partnerships and their transformative potential.

Lingering Challenges

Despite the remarkable achievements of the DGNN and Uganda partnership, several challenges persist, demanding continuous effort and innovation to address. The sustainability of programs remains a pressing concern, as securing ongoing funding and resources is critical to maintaining and expanding the partnership's initiatives. This challenge underscores the need to develop innovative funding models and strengthen local capacity to ensure that progress is preserved and built upon. Expanding access to care continues to be a hurdle, with geographic, economic, and infrastructural barriers limiting the reach of neurosurgical services to remote and underserved populations in Uganda.

Bridging the gap between the need for neurosurgical services and the availability of such services is an ongoing struggle. Despite efforts to expand neurosurgical capacity and access, the demand continues to outpace the supply, highlighting the necessity for further expansion of training programs and health care infrastructure. Moreover, the evolving nature of health care needs and advancements in neurosurgery calls for continuous updates to training curricula and treatment methodologies to ensure that providers are equipped with the latest knowledge and skills. Addressing these lingering challenges requires not only sustained commitment and resources but also a willingness to innovate and adapt to changing circumstances and needs.

To surmount these enduring obstacles, the partnership must continue to foster collaboration with various stakeholders, including government bodies, private sector entities, and community organizations. Developing strategic alliances and leveraging technology can enhance access to care and education. Furthermore, a focus on building local leadership and research capacity is essential for creating self-sustaining systems that can adapt and thrive in the face of challenges. As the partnership progresses, these persistent challenges will serve as focal points for strategic planning and action, driving continued innovation and improvement in global neurosurgery.

Recommendations for Dyad Development

For those inspired to initiate or enhance a dyad partnership in global neurosurgery, the experience of the DGNN and Uganda dyad offers valuable insights and lessons. The foundation of any successful partnership lies in mutual respect and shared goals, establishing a common vision that guides all activities and decisions. This foundation facilitates effective communication and collaboration, ensuring that both partners contribute to and benefit from the partnership. Additionally, respecting each partner's unique contributions, perspectives, and needs fosters an environment of inclusivity and equity, which is essential for long-term success.

Navigating challenges with resilience is another critical recommendation for those embarking on dyad development. The path of international collaboration is inevitably marked by obstacles, ranging from logistical hurdles to cultural misunderstandings. Adopting a resilient and adaptable mindset allows partners to navigate these challenges constructively, viewing them as opportunities for learning and growth rather than insurmountable barriers. This approach also encourages the exploration of innovative solutions and the willingness to pivot strategies in response to evolving circumstances and needs.

Finally, committing to the long-term vision of the partnership is paramount. Sustainable impact requires patience, dedication, and a long-term commitment beyond immediate outcomes. Building strong, enduring relationships with local communities, stakeholders, and institutions is crucial for ensuring the sustainability and scalability of initiatives. Partners should also invest in capacity building and leadership development within the target communities to empower local ownership.

SUMMARY

This article delves into the transformative, dyadic partnership between DGNN and Uganda, highlighting its comprehensive approach toward improving neurosurgical care through service, research, and training. The partnership, characterized by a blend of mutual respect, shared objectives, and a commitment to equity, has led to significant accomplishments, including the saving of countless lives through direct neurosurgical interventions, the establishment of a neurosurgery residency program to address the critical shortage of neurosurgeons, the expansion of neurosurgical services across multiple locations in Uganda, and the initiation of specialized clinics for conditions like epilepsy. Furthermore, the partnership has facilitated extensive training for various health care professionals and produced a wealth of research outputs, substantially contributing to the global body of knowledge in neurosurgery and setting a benchmark for similar initiatives worldwide.

Despite these achievements, the partnership faces ongoing challenges, such as ensuring the sustainability of its programs, expanding access to care, and bridging the gap between the need and availability of services. These challenges underscore the necessity for continuous innovation, collaboration, and strategic planning. Actionable recommendations include the development of effective dyads in global neurosurgery, emphasizing the importance of building on a foundation of mutual respect, navigating challenges with resilience, and committing to a long-term vision. The DGNN and Uganda partnership not only exemplifies the profound impact of international collaborations in addressing global health inequities but also serves as an inspirational model for future endeavors in global neurosurgery.

CALL TO ACTION

As we stand at the crossroads of global health and equity, the DGNN and Uganda partnership illuminates a path forward, showcasing the transformative power of collaboration, innovation, and mutual respect. This partnership has saved and improved countless lives through direct neurosurgical interventions and laid a sustainable foundation for the future through education, research, and capacity building. By expanding neurosurgical services, establishing a neurosurgery residency, and fostering a culture of continuous learning and improvement, this collaboration stands as a beacon of hope and a model for what can be achieved when diverse groups unite toward a common goal. The journey of the DGNN and Uganda partnership, marked by significant accomplishments and ongoing challenges, offers invaluable lessons for the global health community, demonstrating the impact of perseverance, partnership, and shared vision in overcoming global health disparities.

CLINICS CARE POINTS

Pearls

- Establish strong local partnerships: Collaboration with local health care providers and institutions ensures culturally appropriate and sustainable interventions.
- Invest in training and capacity building: Developing local expertise through comprehensive training programs for all levels of health care providers ensures sustainability and scalability of health services, reducing dependency on external support.
- Leverage technology for education and service delivery: Technology and digital learning platforms can significantly enhance access to specialized care and education, especially in remote or underserved areas.
- Adopt a multidisciplinary approach: Integrating services across different health care disciplines promotes comprehensive care, improving patient outcomes.
- Focus on research and data: Conducting local research helps identify specific health needs, monitor outcomes, and guide evidence-based interventions.

Pitfalls

- Underestimating cultural differences: Failing to account for and respect cultural differences can hinder the effectiveness of health interventions and partnerships.
- Ignoring sustainability: Initiatives that do not consider long-term sustainability from the outset risk ending once external support concludes.
- Overlooking local expertise: Not involving local health care providers and experts in the planning and implementation phases can lead to interventions not tailored to the specific context or needs, reducing their effectiveness and acceptance.
- Neglecting comprehensive needs assessment: Initiating projects without a thorough understanding of the local health care landscape, including existing resources and gaps, can lead to redundant efforts or misallocating resources.
- Failing to adapt and innovate: Adhering rigidly to initial plans without considering feedback, monitoring outcomes, and being willing to pivot strategies can prevent dyads from achieving their full potential and addressing evolving health care challenges.

DISCLOSURE

The authors have no relevant disclosures.

REFERENCES

1. Fuller A, Haglund M. The Importance of Collaboration in Global Neurosurgery. Journal of Global Neurosurgery 2021;1(1):78–9. Available at: http://198.12.226.205/index.php/jgn/article/view/238. [Accessed 1 October 2021].
2. Ukachukwu AEK, Seas A, Petitt Z, et al. Assessing the Success and Sustainability of Global Neurosurgery Collaborations: Systematic Review and Adaptation of the Framework for Assessment of InteRNational Surgical Success Criteria. World Neurosurg 2022;167:111–21. https://doi.org/10.1016/j.wneu.2022.08.131.
3. Maleknia P, Shlobin NA, Johnston JM Jr, et al. Establishing collaborations in global neurosurgery: The role of InterSurgeon. J Clin Neurosci 2022;100: 164–8. https://doi.org/10.1016/j.jocn.2022.04.019.
4. Onyia CU, Ojo OA. Collaborative International Neurosurgery Education for Africa–The Journey So Far and the Way Forward. World Neurosurg 2020; 141:e566–75. https://doi.org/10.1016/j.wneu.2020.05.242.
5. Uche EO, Sundblom J, Uko UK, et al. Global neurosurgery over a 60-year period: Conceptual foundations, time reference, emerging Co-ordinates and prospects for collaborative interventions in low and middle income countries. Brain Spine 2022;2: 101187. https://doi.org/10.1016/j.bas.2022.101187.
6. Meara JG, Leather AJM, Hagander L, et al. Global Surgery 2030: evidence and solutions for achieving health, welfare, and economic development. Lancet 2015;386(9993):569–624. https://doi.org/10.1016/S0140-6736(15)60160-X.
7. Dare AJ, Grimes CE, Gillies R, et al. Global surgery: defining an emerging global health field. Lancet

2014;384(9961):2245–7. https://doi.org/10.1016/S0140-6736(14)60237-3.

8. Dempsey RJ. Worldwide Partners in Global Neurosurgery: The Concept of Dyads. In: Dempsey RJ, editor. Global neurosurgery: a reflection from a life in the field. Switzerland: Springer Nature; 2023. p. 73–5. https://doi.org/10.1007/978-3-031-41049-9_21.

9. Dempsey RJ. Twinning of Neurosurgical Educational Programs to Address Resident Future Needs in Global Neurosurgery. Available at: https://www.wfns.org/newsletter/180.

10. Fuller A, Tran T, Muhumuza M, et al. Building neurosurgical capacity in low and middle income countries. eNeurologicalSci 2016;3:1–6. https://doi.org/10.1016/j.ensci.2015.10.003.

11. Haglund MM, Kiryabwire J, Parker S, et al. Surgical capacity building in Uganda through twinning, technology, and training camps. World J Surg 2011;35(6):1175–82. https://doi.org/10.1007/s00268-011-1080-0.

12. Park KB, Johnson WD, Dempsey RJ. Global Neurosurgery: The Unmet Need. World Neurosurg 2016;88:32–5. https://doi.org/10.1016/j.wneu.2015.12.048.

13. Fuller AT, Arraez MA, Haglund MM. The Role of Nonprofit and Academic Institutions in Global Neurosurgery. In: Germano IM, editor. Neurosurgery and global health. Springer International Publishing; 2022. p. 309–24. https://doi.org/10.1007/978-3-030-86656-3_22.

14. Dewan MC, Rattani A, Fieggen G, et al. Global neurosurgery: the current capacity and deficit in the provision of essential neurosurgical care. Executive Summary of the Global Neurosurgery Initiative at the Program in Global Surgery and Social Change. J Neurosurg 2018;1–10. https://doi.org/10.3171/2017.11.JNS171500.

15. Dewan MC, Rattani A, Gupta S, et al. Estimating the global incidence of traumatic brain injury. J Neurosurg 2018;1–18. https://doi.org/10.3171/2017.10.JNS17352.

16. Tran TM, Fuller AT, Kiryabwire J, et al. Distribution and characteristics of severe traumatic brain injury at Mulago National Referral Hospital in Uganda. World Neurosurg 2015;83(3):269–77. https://doi.org/10.1016/j.wneu.2014.12.028.

17. Butler EK, Tran TM, Nagarajan N, et al. Epidemiology of pediatric surgical needs in low-income countries. PLoS One 2017;12(3):e0170968. https://doi.org/10.1371/journal.pone.0170968.

18. Fuller AT, Corley J, Tran TM, et al. Prevalence of Surgically Untreated Face, Head, and Neck Conditions in Uganda: A Cross-Sectional Nationwide Household Survey. World Neurosurg 2018;110:e747–54. https://doi.org/10.1016/j.wneu.2017.11.099.

19. Farber SH, Vissoci JRN, Tran TM, et al. Geospatial Analysis of Unmet Surgical Need in Uganda: An Analysis of SOSAS Survey Data. World J Surg 2017;41(2):353–63. https://doi.org/10.1007/s00268-016-3689-5.

20. Tran TM, Farber SH, Vissoci JR, et al. Geographic access and relationship to unmet surgical need in Uganda: a geospatial analysis of a household survey on burden of surgical conditions in Uganda. Annals of Global Health 2016;82(3):564–5.

21. Haglund MM, Warf B, Fuller A, et al. Past, Present, and Future of Neurosurgery in Uganda. Neurosurgery 2017;80(4):656–61. https://doi.org/10.1093/neuros/nyw159.

22. Fuller AT, Haglund MM, Lim S, et al. Pediatric Neurosurgical Outcomes Following a Neurosurgery Health System Intervention at Mulago National Referral Hospital in Uganda. World Neurosurg 2016;95:309–14. https://doi.org/10.1016/j.wneu.2016.07.090.

23. Paradie E, Warman PI, Waguia-Kouam R, et al. The Scope, Growth, and Inequities of the Global Neurosurgery Literature: A Bibliometric Analysis. World Neurosurg 2022;167:e670–84. https://doi.org/10.1016/j.wneu.2022.08.074.

24. Kitya D, Najjuma JN, Punchak M, et al. Outcomes at discharge of pediatric traumatic brain injury (pTBI) in Western Uganda: a prospective cohort study. J Glob Neurosurg 2022.

25. Adil SM, Elahi C, Patel DN, et al. Deep Learning to Predict Traumatic Brain Injury Outcomes in the Low-Resource Setting. World Neurosurg 2022;164:e8–16. https://doi.org/10.1016/j.wneu.2022.02.097.

26. Nwosu C, Batakana S, Vissoci J, et al. Identifying the needs and barriers to patient-family education to design educational interventions that will improve neurosurgery patient outcomes in Mulago hospital, Uganda. Ann Glob Health 2017;83(1):123. https://doi.org/10.1016/j.aogh.2017.03.275.

27. Kuo BJ, Vaca SD, Vissoci JRN, et al. A prospective neurosurgical registry evaluating the clinical care of traumatic brain injury patients presenting to Mulago National Referral Hospital in Uganda. PLoS One 2017;12(10):e0182285. https://doi.org/10.1371/journal.pone.0182285.

28. Lu Z, Tshimbombu TN, Abu-Bonsrah N, et al. Transnational Capacity Building Efforts in Global Neurosurgery: A Review and Analysis of Their Impact and Determinants of Success. World Neurosurg 2023;173:188–98. https://doi.org/10.1016/j.wneu.2023.01.120. e3.

29. Ukachukwu AEK, Still MEH, Seas A, et al. Fulfilling the specialist neurosurgical workforce needs in Africa: a systematic review and projection toward 2030. J Neurosurg 2023;138(4):1102–13. https://doi.org/10.3171/2022.2.JNS211984.

30. Ramasubramanian P, Prose N, Johnson T, et al. "Walking the Journey Together": Creating a unique learning module in provider-patient communication for the care of epilepsy in Uganda. Epilepsy Behav

2023;140:109096.   https://doi.org/10.1016/j.yebeh.
2023.109096.

31. Arinda A, Ouma S, Kalani K, et al. Evaluation of a
tailored epilepsy training program for healthcare providers in Uganda. Epilepsy Behav 2023;138:108977.
https://doi.org/10.1016/j.yebeh.2022.108977.

32. Koltai DC, Smith CE, Cai GY, et al. Healthcare provider perspectives regarding epilepsy care in
Uganda. Epilepsy Behav 2020;107294. https://doi.
org/10.1016/j.yebeh.2020.107294.

33. Karekezi C, El Khamlichi A, El Ouahabi A, et al. The
impact of African-trained neurosurgeons on sub-
Saharan Africa. Neurosurg Focus 2020;48(3):E4.
https://doi.org/10.3171/2019.12.FOCUS19853.

34. El Khamlichi A. African neurosurgery: current situation, priorities, and needs. Neurosurgery 2001;
48(6):1344–7.   https://doi.org/10.1097/00006123-
200106000-00034.

35. El Khamlichi A. Neurosurgery in Africa. Clin Neurosurg 2005;52:214–7. Available at: https://www.ncbi.
nlm.nih.gov/pubmed/16626073.

36. Fuller AT, Almojuela A, Kaddumukasa MN, et al.
Hospital-based epilepsy care in Uganda: A prospective study of three major public referral hospitals. Epilepsy Behav 2020;107301. https://doi.org/
10.1016/j.yebeh.2020.107301.

37. Namusisi J, Kyoyagala S, Nantongo J, et al. Poor
seizure control among children attending a tertiary
hospital in south western Uganda - A retrospective
study. Int J Gen Med 2023;16:895–904. https://doi.
org/10.2147/IJGM.S398318.

38. Jane N, Mike K, Stephen S, et al. Poor seizure control
among children attending a tertiary hospital in South
Western Uganda- a retrospective study. Int J Gen
Med 2023. https://doi.org/10.2147/IJGM.S398318.

Education and Training in Global Neurosurgery
Current State and Path Toward a Uniform Curriculum

Nathan A. Shlobin, MD, MBA[a],*, Yosef Ellenbogen, MD[b],
Mojgan Hodaie, MD[b,c,d], Gail Rosseau, MD[e,f]

KEYWORDS

- Global health • Global surgery • Health care disparities • Medical training • Neurologic surgery
- Neurosurgical disease • Residency

KEY POINTS

- Few opportunities for neurosurgical training may exist in low-income and middle-income countries.
- Core components of neurosurgical training are defined.
- A gold standard for neurosurgical training is necessary to ensure a comprehensive training experience, albeit applied in contextually appropriate manner.

INTRODUCTION

Annually, approximately 22.6 million patients suffer from neurologic disorders or injuries requiring neurosurgical consultation, including 13.8 million who require surgery.[1] Approximately 23,300 additional neurosurgeons are needed to cover more than 5 million essential neurosurgical cases that are unmet each year, all of which occur in low-income and middle-income countries (LMICs).[1] The field of global neurosurgery arose at the intersection of neurosurgery and public health to address this unmet need through clinical practice, research, advocacy, and education.[2–4] Although previously commonly utilized to address the global burden of neurosurgical disease, mission trips are unable to provide long-term solutions due to limited follow-up after the missions from the external team and a lack of training of local health care personnel to manage complex neurosurgical conditions.[5] Instead, education and training has been recognized as a sustainable measure to increase neurosurgical capacity by empowering local populations.[5] In this manuscript, we describe current education and training in neurosurgery to characterize the landscape of neurosurgical training worldwide, as well as novel educational mechanisms that have emerged in recent years. Then, we synthesize a uniform educational curriculum to provide

^a Department of Neurosurgery, Neurological Institute of New York, New York Presbyterian Hospital - Columbia University Irving Medical Center, 710 West 168th Street, 4th Floor, New York, NY 10032, USA; ^b Division of Neurosurgery, Department of Surgery, University of Toronto, Stewart Building 149 College Street, 5th Floor, Toronto, ON M5T 1P5, Canada; ^c Division of Brain, Imaging & Behaviour, Krembil Research Institute, University Health Network, 60 Leonard Avenue, Toronto, ON M5T 0S8, Canada; ^d Institute of Medical Science, Temerty Faculty of Medicine, University of Toronto, Medical Sciences Building, 1 King's College Cir, Toronto, ON M5S 1A8, Canada; ^e Department of Neurological Surgery, George Washington University School of Medicine and Health Sciences, 2150 Pennsylvania Avenue, NW, Suite 7-420, Washington, DC 20037, USA; ^f Barrow Global, Barrow Neurological Institute, 2910 N 3rd Avenue, Phoenix, AZ 85013, USA

* Corresponding author. 676 North St. Clair Street, Suite 2210, Chicago, IL 60611.

E-mail address: nshlobin@gmail.com

Twitter: @NathanShlobin (N.A.S.); @YosefEllenbogen (Y.E.); @mhodaie (M.H.); @grosseaumd (G.R.)

Neurosurg Clin N Am 35 (2024) 429–437
https://doi.org/10.1016/j.nec.2024.05.005
1042-3680/24/© 2024 Elsevier Inc. All rights are reserved, including those for text and data mining, AI training, and similar technologies.

a gold standard for neurosurgical care and a context-specific pathway for achieving this standard. It is our hope that this manuscript will guide the development of local training programs adapted to local political, economic, social, cultural, and linguistic realities.

DISCUSSION
Current State of Education and Training in Neurosurgery

High-income countries

Current education and training pathways in neurosurgery differ in significant ways based on location. In general, neurosurgery residency programs in high-income countries (HICs) are accredited by a national governing body that stipulates basic requirements for all residency programs in the country.[6] In the United States, neurosurgical residency is 7 years long, involving an intern year that may be neurosurgery-focused or general, 2 to 3 years of junior residency, 1 to 2 years of research, and 1 to 2 senior years. However, the postgraduate year 7 has increasingly been utilized for enfolded fellowships or as a transition-to-practice year.[7] All residency training is governed by the Accreditation Council for Graduate Medical Education (ACGME), which has instituted a 80-h limit on work hours per week.[6] Average graduating case volumes are approximately 1600 cases, albeit with high variability between programs.[8–10] Although the number of cases performed per faculty is associated with resident case volume, the program case volume, number of operating attending neurosurgeons, number of residents, number of research years, or presence of fellows are not.[10] In Canada, neurosurgery residency is 6 years, consisting of a general intern year, 3 years of junior residency, 1 research year, and 2 years of senior residency. There is an opportunity for residents to extend their training during residency and undertake a graduate degree through the establishment of the Surgeon-Scientist Training Programs.[11] There is an average of 1845 neurosurgical cases performed per residency program.[12] Neurosurgery residency programs are accredited by the Royal College of Physicians and Surgeons in Canada.[10] In Australia and New Zealand, progression through training is competency-based, rather than based on time.[13] In general, training is 5 to 7 years, involving basic modules for 1 to 2 years, intermediate modules for 3 years, and advanced modules for 1 to 2 years, with a requirement that residents must move away from their home state at least once to diversify their experience.[13] Most residents complete training in 5 to 6 years.[14] Training programs are accredited by the Neurosurgical Society of Australasia every 5 years.[13] In contrast, residency training in Europe is not as standardized, with training ranging from 4 to 6 years.[15] Although the European Association of Neurologic Societies (EANS) has guidelines for residency, each country has its own board requirements and neurosurgical curriculum.[16] Theoretic and practical aspects of training are highly variable.[17] Although a 48-h work-week has been implemented through the European Working Time directive, most training programs do not adhere to this directive.[18,19] A recent survey of neurosurgeons from nearly all EANS member states indicated that 80.2% of neurosurgeons believed that a joint standardized neurosurgical certificate in Europe is necessary.[20] The mean number of surgical procedures participated in during residency was 1594.[21,22] Residency programs in HICs typically include a combination of operating room-based training, cadaver laboratories, didactics, research mentorship, and journal clubs. Simulation training, including boot camps, has also been increasingly incorporated into all HIC programs.[23,24]

Low-income and middle-income countries

There are challenges to medical education in areas where access to health care is limited. Some LMICs do not have neurosurgery residency programs, requiring potential residents to move abroad to train.[25] Typically, a few LMICs train a large proportion of LMIC neurosurgeons. Large regional programs include Recife, Brazil, and Rabat, Morocco, via the World Federation of Neurosurgical Societies (WFNS) Rabat Training Center, which also provided to additional programs in African through the Africa 100 program.[26,27] Additional WFNS Reference Centers worldwide have been approved to offer training based on a review of their curriculum, but centralized funding for these programs is generally not available. Approximately 26.2% of trainees have to pay tuition for their neurosurgical training and do not receive a salary, a significantly higher proportion relative to HICs.[28] Many individuals are deterred from pursuing a career in neurosurgery due to a lack of resources. Those who pay, encounter considerable financial strain, often forcing them to work additional shifts to pay for this tuition or leave the residency program if they are unable to continue paying. The World Bank has insisted that countries receiving debt restructuring assistance utilize austerity measures in their federal budgeting, forcing them to reduce their workforce or hours of employment, including for health care workers.[29,30] Individuals often spend a few years in general surgery without learning neurosurgical skills.[31] Neurosurgical training is 2 to 3 years in some LMICs.[31]

Coupled with low operative time, these factors underscore the perceived inadequacy of operative training. In one survey, over 60% of residents reported limited hands-on training and insufficient exposure to emergent subspecialties.[32] Another survey found that subspecialty training is less available to trainees in LMICs than HICs.[25] Residents often learn as apprentices, leaving them with limited training opportunities. These factors result in a vicious cycle in which inadequate training may discourage neurosurgeons from performing certain types of cases, leading to deficiencies once the next generation of neurosurgeons. Similarly, didactic courses and cadaver laboratories are often unavailable,[33,34] limiting complementary learning opportunities to operative training. Research and mentorship opportunities are also often lacking.[33]

In total, these deficiencies lead neurosurgical trainees in LMICs to believe that they are unprepared. A survey in Sub-Saharan Africa indicated that only 37% of respondents reported that their training program adequately prepared them to address neurosurgical cases.[35] Respondents cited a lack of physical resources, practical workshops, program structure, and topic-specific lectures.[35] Additionally, surveys have indicated greater work hours in LMICs and a concern about inadequate work hour regulations,[25,32] highlighting that many activities that residents in LMICs perform may not be educational.

It is important to qualify these deficiencies by noting that some LMIC environments provide strong clinical training. Some LMICs, such as Brazil, have a well-developed neurosurgical training infrastructure but too few neurosurgeons, allowing neurosurgical trainees the opportunity to become involved in complex cases and augment their surgical skills. Moreover, certain types of cases are more common in LMICs than HICs. Some LMICs lack access to angiography suites or equipment for endovascular interventions. As a result, open cerebrovascular neurosurgery is performed more frequently than in many centers in HICs.[36,37] Additionally, the success of folic acid fortification in HICs has reduced the incidence of spina bifida such that neurosurgical trainees in HICs gain little experience in myelomeningocele repair during residency and may travel to LMICs to gain greater exposure.[38,39]

As a result of the limitations seen in most resource-constrained settings, neurosurgeons in these countries must often fend for themselves to gain a comprehensive training experience. Innovative disruption in global neurosurgery has involved teaching oneself. Although teaching oneself may be a powerful educational tool, it cannot substitute entirely for deliberate guidance and instruction. Systems-based suggestions for improvement of neurosurgical training in LMICs include the creation of a robust network of international collaboration for reciprocal certification, skills sharing, and subspecialty training; incorporation of in-serve residency and fellowship within a framework of expanding access to neurosurgical care; and engaging in health systems strengthening and infrastructure development.[40]

Novel Educational Mechanisms

In addition to standard neurosurgery residency programs, novel educational mechanisms have emerged. One is establishing residency programs in countries lacking training programs. The College of Surgeons of Southern, Eastern, and Central Africa has worked with neurosurgeons to develop neurosurgical training and accreditation. The Duke Neurosurgery East Africa Project in Uganda has created a residency program in Uganda to train local neurosurgeons.[41–43] Project Medishare: Haiti has developed a self-sustaining neurosurgical residency program in Haiti with sponsorship of the Haitian Ministry of Health and National Medical School and provided sustainable health care and community development services.[42,44] The Barrow Global program of Barrow Neurologic Institute is working with Kilimanjaro Christian Medical Center to develop a residency program in northern Tanzania. With the support of the Global Neurosurgery Committee, the first 2 trainees from Sierra Leone are training in Morocco, with a sustainability plan in place to support their practice when they return to their native countries after training.

Another is "twinning" programs between a well-experienced and emerging institution. The Foundation for International Education in Neurologic Surgery utilizes an approach of "service through education" to train neurosurgeons and develop local residency programs.[45] The Clack Family fellowship support the training of neurosurgeons in countries where they are completing their training, while the Bassett fellowships allow neurosurgeons from LMICs to travel to training programs in North America for 3 months of focused training.[46] Additionally, the Weill Cornell Neurosurgery-Tanzania Collaboration involves reciprocal fellowships between Weill Cornell and the Muhimbili Orthopedic Institute to facilitate training, annual didactics, and a weekly remote case review.[42,47] The Children's Hospital of Alabama-Vietnam partnership consists of in-country targeted hands on-training in Vietnam, out-of-country fellowship training at the Children's Hospital of Alabama, and ongoing mentorship using virtual interactive presence technologies to provide real-time targeted feedback during surgical case livestreams.[48,49] The Co-Pilot project involves international fellowships for Ukrainian neurosurgeons, cadaveric neuroanatomy courses, and educational conferences between American and Ukrainian neurosurgeons.[50] The International Neurosurgical Twinning Model for Africa from the Swedish African Neurosurgical Collaboration is a 5 phase model involving an initial professional linkage, justification visit, philanthropic travel, targeted benevolent donation, and focused clinical partnership.[51]

Other models also exist. The Spanish-Based Neurosurgery Education and Development Foundation employs a simultaneous tripartite model, each with multiple levels.[52–54] The logic behind this model is that interventions become more complex at each level of development as the local team gains greater capability and capacity to provide neurosurgical care.[53] The "Equip" principle signifies assistance for local neurosurgeons in acquiring infrastructure, while "Treat" is providing direct medical care. The "Train" principle refers to mentoring, then residency program accreditation, and finally continuous training of future generations of neurosurgeons by neurosurgeons trained in this model.[53]

Most existing models involve collaborations between HIC and LMIC partners.[55] Unfortunately, LMIC-LMIC collaborations for neurosurgical training are rare due to inadequate funding or coordination difficulties. However, collaborations between HICs and LMICs may encounter pitfalls, including a lack of attention to local needs and priorities, insufficient involvement of local personnel, inadequate coordination with local and national governments, initiatives with limited or short-term impact, and the potential for exploitation. HIC-LMIC collaborations must seek to develop sustainable and equitable training initiatives based on local needs and priorities and aimed at increasing the capability of local physicians and health care personnel to provide neurosurgical care. As in research collaborations, the goal of training partnerships between HICs and LMICs must be to promote LMIC independence and growth.[56]

Neurosurgeons have developed symposiums to determine best practices for neurosurgical training. "Global Neurosurgery 2019: A Practical Symposium" sought to centralize resources and converge parallel efforts in neurosurgical education.[42] The Global Neurosurgery Education Summit in 2021 aimed to identify factors for success in improving access, equity, and quality in clinical global neurosurgery training fellowships.[57] Hybrid fellowships with in-person operative teaching, didactics employing a flipped classroom approach for topics such as patient selection and anatomy, and remote narration of operative procedures with stop-action questioning and discussion gained reasonable support among attendees of this summit.[57] Additionally, there has been a push toward integration of targeted public health education in neurosurgical training in LMICs and HICs.[58]

Components of a Neurosurgical Training Curriculum

Neurosurgical training demands a deep understanding of anatomy, physiology, and operative skills to safely and independently care for patients with neurosurgical pathologies.[59] While the components of neurosurgical training curricula may differ regionally and adapt to local health systems, the ultimate goal is consistent: to produce capable neurosurgeons. These variations can affect the length of training, the responsibilities assigned to residents, the balance between didactic and hands-on surgical experience, and the criteria for evaluating trainees.[60] These differences stem from the interplay among stakeholders and the logistical challenges inherent in regional training differences.[16,35] **Fig. 1** outlines key components of neurosurgical training.

The cornerstone in a neurosurgical training curriculum consists of the operative room experience. This is an area of training that consists of direct hands-on experiential learning under the guidance of a staff surgeon.[61,62] This apprenticeship-style component can vary significantly between educators, programs, and countries, hinging on the development of trust between the mentor and the trainee. Given the importance of hands-on surgical experience in the training of a surgeon, there have been efforts to standardize this component of the surgical curriculum. One such effort has been through instituting a minimum number of cases required per a specific operation. This has

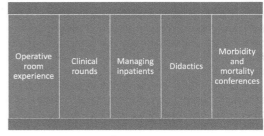

Fig. 1. Components of neurosurgical training.

been implemented as a standard in several countries, such as the United States through the ACGME as in Canada through the Royal College of Physicians and Surgeons of Canada (RCPSC). The ACGME implemented a minimum number of cases as the "lead surgeon" in order to graduate in 2019.[63] The uptake of this method is somewhat varied and studies have demonstrated there is a variable degree inaccurate and underestimation of cases performed using this method.[64,65] The RCPSC has initiated a similar approach with the Competency by Design curriculum (CBD) which spans all medical and surgical specialities.[66] This effort was initiated in 2017 and adopted by all surgical training programs in Canada by 2019.[67] This CBD curriculum formalizes and standardizes the surgical experience by requiring an Entrusted Professional Encounter (EPA) evaluation to be conducted after each surgical procedure with a pre-defined number of EPAs that require completion at each stage of residency training. While implementation varies, the principle of case log tracking remains a useful tool for standardization within neurosurgical training centers.[68]

In addition to operative experience, the educational value of clinical rounds and managing an inpatient neurosurgical service cannot be understated. These embedded clinical experiences within a residency curriculum may be thought of as "silently" educational but serve a critical role in providing trainees with the requisite experience to develop clinical acumen and an in-depth understanding of the natural history of neurosurgical diseases. This in turn helps trainees with decision making regarding operative and non-operative management of neurosurgical patients. Though critical to the curriculum of a neurosurgical curriculum, this component of the training is contextual to the local environment and health system and thus may vary in structure between programs. The didactic component of the neurosurgical curriculum also plays a vital role in resident education and supplements the clinical and surgical curriculum that enables residents to integrate contemporary neurosurgical practice with foundational knowledge. This is often characterized by a dedicated lectureship (termed "educational rounds") led by surgical staff and multidisciplinary groups.[69] This component of the surgical curriculum has been associated with a significant improvement in resident satisfaction.[70] Additionally, this is an opportunity for collaboration among multiple training programs, where resources can be pooled and larger programs can supplement programs in mid and low-income countries.[35,71]

Another component of neurosurgical training is Morbidity and Mortality (M and M) conferences.

These serve as a platform for collective learning from outcomes, fostering a culture where patient safety and quality improvement are paramount.[72] Case presentations and reviews within a collaborative educational setting encourage critical thinking and peer-to-peer learning. Such interactions are pivotal in developing a resident's ability to articulate and defend clinical reasoning. Kashiwazaki and colleagues demonstrated that the M and M rounds served to tangibly reduce the number of "avoidable" complications within a 5-year study period.[73] This is a potential area where teleconferences and "Twinning" programs can serve to supplement the educational value of this in smaller and lower resource settings.[45]

Evaluation and Examinations

The evaluation of residents lacks universal standardization and thus, these processes are governed on a local level. While there exists regional variation in this regard, there is an increasing movement toward more frequent evaluations to be conducted.[74] This has been particularly notable in countries that have adopted competency-based medical education, such as the United States, Canada, Australia, Denmark, and Switzerland.[75] However, the many intangible components of neurosurgical training as well as local practice variations make uniform evaluation criteria challenging. Similarly, the components of credentialing and licensing residents to independent staff also experiences significant variations in different countries.[59] Though widespread standardization of the credentialing process may pose significant logistical challenges due to different health systems and governing bodies, there is an interest in harmonizing these processes in certain locations, such as in Europe.[20]

Toward a "Gold" Standard

The need for a high standard of neurosurgical care is universal and applicable to patients globally. However, the varied nature of health systems and their impact on neurosurgical care necessitates a tailored approach that considers the specific limitations and strengths of each educational setting.[1,4,76] Though the components of a neurosurgery curriculum are similar across different training programs, the degree to which each aspect of the curriculum is represented and to how it may be implemented differs. There is a need to establish a high standard of care to all patients with neurosurgical pathologies regardless of country or socioeconomic status. A cross-sectional survey of the Young Neurosurgeons Forum consisting of 91 neurosurgeons practicing in Latin America and Caribbean found that most respondents cited a lack of standardized curriculum was a significant barrier in their training and practice.[77] This underscores the need for a "gold" standard in neurosurgery residency curriculum. However, the complex interplay of how different health systems influence neurosurgical care delivery necessitates a personalized approach that invokes practical limitations and advantages of each training environment. Outlining these pathways is crucial for setting a universal benchmark that can be aspired to globally.[35,78]

Though a neurosurgery curriculum can take shape in multiple ways, the importance of an established pre-specified curriculum with tangible milestones, evaluations, and checkpoints laid out a priori is crucial. This serves as an "educational contract" whereby the local institution and resident trainee can align expectations and provide a skeleton framework. An educational contract represents a tangible commitment to this uniform standard, detailing explicit responsibilities for both the resident and the institution. It is a mechanism for accountability, ensuring that the objectives of the educational curriculum are met.

SUMMARY

The objective of neurosurgical training curricula is to achieve consistency in the outcomes of trainees, ensuring they can competently address neurosurgical pathologies. The core elements of training—operative experience, academic study, patient management, and outcome analysis—differ by region but are bound by this common goal. Educational contracts serve to formalize this aim, setting clear expectations and responsibilities for both the trainee and the institution. While the route to standardized outcomes is challenged by variations in health care systems and educational environments, the drive for a uniform standard in trainee competency underscores the commitment to quality patient care across the globe.

CLINICS CARE POINTS

- Low- and middle-income countries lack access to neurosurgical training opportunities.
- Residency programs should be contextually appropriate.

DISCLOSURES

The authors have nothing to disclose.

REFERENCES

1. Dewan MC, Rattani A, Fieggen G, et al. Global neurosurgery: the current capacity and deficit in the provision of essential neurosurgical care. Executive Summary of the Global Neurosurgery Initiative at the Program in Global Surgery and Social Change. J Neurosurg 2018;130(4):1055–64.
2. Park KB, Johnson WD, Dempsey RJ. Global neurosurgery: the unmet need. World neurosurgery 2016;88:32–5.
3. Haglund MM, Fuller AT. Global neurosurgery: innovators, strategies, and the way forward: JNSPG 75th Anniversary Invited Review Article. J Neurosurg 2019; 131(4):993–9.
4. Niquen-Jimenez M, Wishart D, Garcia RM, et al. A bibliographic analysis of the most cited articles in global neurosurgery. World neurosurgery 2020; 144:e195–203.
5. Dempsey RJ, Buckley NA. Education-based solutions to the global burden of neurosurgical disease. World neurosurgery 2020;140:e1–6.
6. Fargen KM, Chakraborty A, Friedman WA. Results of a national neurosurgery resident survey on duty hour regulations. Neurosurgery 2011;69(6):1162–70.
7. Kolcun JPG, Mazza JM, Pawlowski KD, et al. The evolving role of postgraduate year 7 in neurological surgery residency. Neurosurgery 2024;94(2): 350–7.
8. Agarwal N, White MD, Cohen J, et al. Longitudinal survey of cranial case log entries during neurological surgery residency training. J Neurosurg 2018; 130(6):2025–31.
9. Hopkins BS, Shlobin NA, Kesavabhotla K, et al. Case volume analysis of neurological surgery training programs in the United States: 2017-2019. Neurosurgery Open 2021;2(1):okaa017.
10. Burkhardt E, Adeeb N, Terrell D, et al. Factors impacting neurosurgery residents' operative case volume: a nationwide survey. J Neurosurg 2023;1(aop): 1–6.
11. McLeod R, Keshavjee S, Ahmed N, et al. History of the Department of Surgery at the University of Toronto: celebrating a centennial of progress and innovation. Can J Surg 2022;65(1):E56.
12. Tso MK, Dakson A, Ahmed SU, et al. Operative landscape at Canadian neurosurgery residency programs. Can J Neurol Sci 2017;44(4):415–9.
13. McAlpine H, Mee E, Laidlaw J, et al. Neurosurgery Education Around the World: Australasia. Neurosurgery and Global Health 2022;209–28.
14. Drummond KJ, Hunn BH, McAlpine HE, et al. Challenges in the Australasian neurosurgery training program: who should be trained and where should they train? Neurosurg Focus 2020;48(3):E10.
15. Ruparelia J, Khatri D, Gosal JS. Duration of Neurosurgery Residency in India and its Impact on

Training: A Comparison of Residency Structures. World Neurosurgery 2021;154:29–31.

16. Burkhardt J-K, Zinn PO, Bozinov O, et al. Neurosurgical education in Europe and the United States of America. Neurosurg Rev 2010;33:409–17.

17. Stienen MN, Netuka D, Demetriades AK, et al. Neurosurgical resident education in Europe—results of a multinational survey. Acta Neurochir 2016;158: 3–15.

18. Schaller K. Neurosurgical training under European law. Acta Neurochir 2013;155:547.

19. Stienen MN, Netuka D, Demetriades AK, et al. Working time of neurosurgical residents in Europe—results of a multinational survey. Acta Neurochir 2016;158:17–25.

20. Navarro R, Mehigan B, Marchesini N, et al. Neurosurgical training and education–General European certification is supported: Results of an EANS survey. Brain and Spine 2023;3:102666.

21. Stienen MN, Freyschlag CF, Schaller K, et al. Procedures performed during neurosurgery residency in Europe. Acta Neurochir 2020;162:2303–11.

22. Stienen MN, Bartek J, Czabanka MA, et al. Neurosurgical procedures performed during residency in Europe—preliminary numbers and time trends. Acta Neurochir 2019;161:843–53.

23. Kilbourn KJ, Leclair NK, Martin JE, et al. Incorporating simulation into the neurosurgical residency curriculum: a program director survey. J Neurosurg 2023;1(aop):1–6.

24. Ganju A, Aoun SG, Daou MR, et al. The role of simulation in neurosurgical education: a survey of 99 United States neurosurgery program directors. World neurosurgery 2013;80(5):e1–8.

25. Sarpong K, Fadalla T, Garba DL, et al. Access to training in neurosurgery (Part 1): Global perspectives and contributing factors of barriers to access. Brain and Spine 2022;2:100900.

26. El Khamlichi A. The World Federation of Neurosurgical Societies Rabat Reference Center for training African neurosurgeons: an experience worthy of duplication. World neurosurgery 2014; 81(2):234–9.

27. Karekezi C, El Khamlichi A. Takeoff of African neurosurgery and the world federation of neurosurgical societies rabat training center alumni. World neurosurgery 2019;126:576–80.

28. Garba DL, Fadalla T, Sarpong K, et al. Access to training in neurosurgery (Part 2): The costs of pursuing neurosurgical training. Brain and Spine 2022;2: 100927.

29. Williams D, Thomas S. The impact of austerity on the health workforce and the achievement of human resources for health policies in Ireland (2008–2014). Hum Resour Health 2017;15(1):1–8.

30. Ruckert A, Labonté R, Parker RH. Global healthcare policy and the austerity agenda. The Palgrave International Handbook of Healthcare Policy and Governance 2015;37–53.

31. Kato Y, Liew B, Sufianov A, et al. Review of global neurosurgery education: horizon of neurosurgery in the developing countries. Chinese Neurosurgical Journal 2020;6(03):178–90.

32. Deora H, Garg K, Tripathi M, et al. Residency perception survey among neurosurgery residents in lower-middle-income countries: grassroots evaluation of neurosurgery education. Neurosurg Focus 2020;48(3):E11.

33. Murguia-Fuentes R, Husein N, Vega A, et al. Neurosurgical residency training in Latin America: current status, challenges, and future opportunities. World neurosurgery 2018;120:e1079–97.

34. Gnanakumar S, Bourquin BAEE, Robertson FC, et al. The world federation of neurosurgical Societies young neurosurgeons survey (Part I): demographics, resources, and education. World neurosurgery: X 2020;8:100083.

35. Sader E, Yee P, Hodaie M. Barriers to neurosurgical training in Sub-Saharan Africa: the need for a phased approach to global surgery efforts to improve neurosurgical care. World Neurosurgery 2017;98:397–402.

36. Dokponou YCH, Alihonou T, de Paule Adjiou DKF, et al. Surgical aneurysm repair of aneurysmal subarachnoid hemorrhage in Sub-Saharan Africa: The state of training and management. World Neurosurgery 2023. https://doi.org/10.1016/j.wneu.2023.05.085.

37. Waterkeyn F, Lohkamp L-N, Ikwuegbuenyi CA, et al. Current Treatment Management of Aneurysmal Subarachnoid Hemorrhage with Prevailing Trends and Results in Tanzania: A Single-Center Experience at Muhimbili Orthopedic and Neurosurgery Institute. World Neurosurgery 2023;170:e256–63.

38. Shlobin NA, Roach JT, Kancherla V, et al. The role of neurosurgeons in global public health: the case of folic acid fortification of staple foods to prevent spina bifida. J Neurosurg Pediatr 2022;1(aop):1–8.

39. Gandy K, Castillo H, Rocque BG, et al. Neurosurgical training and global health education: systematic review of challenges and benefits of in-country programs in the care of neural tube defects. Neurosurg Focus 2020;48(3):E14.

40. Ferraris KP, Matsumura H, Wardhana DPW, et al. The state of neurosurgical training and education in East Asia: analysis and strategy development for this frontier of the world. Neurosurg Focus 2020;48(3):E7.

41. Budohoski KP, Ngerageza JG, Austard B, et al. Neurosurgery in East Africa: innovations. World neurosurgery 2018;113:436–52.

42. Schmidt FA, Kirnaz S, Wipplinger C, et al. Review of the highlights from the first annual global neurosurgery 2019: A practical symposium. World Neurosurgery 2020;137:46–54.

43. Fuller A, Tran T, Muhumuza M, et al. Building neurosurgical capacity in low and middle income countries. Eneurologicalsci 2016;3:1–6.

44. Shah AH, Barthélemy E, Lafortune Y, et al. Bridging the gap: creating a self-sustaining neurosurgical residency program in Haiti. Neurosurg Focus 2018; 45(4):E4.

45. Dempsey RJ. Global neurosurgery: the role of the individual neurosurgeon, the Foundation for International Education in Neurological Surgery, and "service through education" to address worldwide need. Neurosurg Focus 2018;45(4):E19.

46. Kanmounye US, Shlobin NA, Dempsey RJ, et al. Foundation for international education in neurosurgery: the next half-century of service through education. Journal of Global Neurosurgery 2021;1(1):68–72.

47. Coburger J, Leng LZ, Rubin DG, et al. Multi-institutional neurosurgical training initiative at a tertiary referral center in Mwanza, Tanzania: where we are after 2 years. World neurosurgery 2014;82(1–2): e1–8.

48. Haji FA, Lepard JR, Davis MC, et al. A model for global surgical training and capacity development: the Children's of Alabama–Viet Nam pediatric neurosurgery partnership. Child's Nerv Syst 2021;37: 627–36.

49. Davis MC, Can DD, Pindrik J, et al. Virtual interactive presence in global surgical education: international collaboration through augmented reality. World neurosurgery 2016;86:103–11.

50. Tomycz LD, Markosian C, Kurilets Sr I, et al. The Co-Pilot Project: an international neurosurgical collaboration in Ukraine. World Neurosurgery 2021;147: e491–515.

51. Uche EO, Mezue WC, Ajuzieogu O, et al. Improving capacity and access to neurosurgery in sub-Saharan Africa using a twinning paradigm pioneered by the Swedish African Neurosurgical Collaboration. Acta Neurochir 2020;162:973–81.

52. Leidinger A, Piquer J, Kim EE, et al. Treating pediatric hydrocephalus at the Neurosurgery Education and Development Institute: the reality in the Zanzibar Archipelago, Tanzania. World Neurosurgery 2018;117:e450–6.

53. Rodríguez-Mena R, Piquer-Martínez J, Llácer-Ortega JL, et al. The NED foundation experience: A model of global neurosurgery. Brain and Spine 2023;3:101741.

54. Leidinger A, Extremera P, Kim EE, et al. The challenges and opportunities of global neurosurgery in East Africa: the Neurosurgery Education and Development model. Neurosurg Focus 2018; 45(4):E8.

55. Paradie E, Warman PI, Waguia-Kouam R, et al. The scope, growth, and inequities of the global neurosurgery literature: a bibliometric analysis. World Neurosurgery 2022;167:e670–84.

56. Ukachukwu A-EK, Seas A, Petitt Z, et al. Assessing the Success and Sustainability of Global Neurosurgery Collaborations: Systematic Review and Adaptation of the Framework for Assessment of InteRNational Surgical Success Criteria. World Neurosurgery 2022;167:111–21.

57. Hoffman C, Härtl R, Shlobin NA, et al. Future directions for global clinical neurosurgical training: challenges and opportunities. World neurosurgery 2022;166:e404–18.

58. Rallo MS, Strong MJ, Teton ZE, et al. Targeted public health training for neurosurgeons: an essential task for the prioritization of neurosurgery in the evolving global health landscape. Neurosurgery 2023;92(1): 10–7.

59. Pieters TA, Susa S, Agarwal N, et al. Credentialing, Certification, and Peer Review Essentials for the Neurosurgeon. World Neurosurgery 2021;151: 364–9.

60. Yaeger KA, Munich SA, Byrne RW, et al. Trends in United States neurosurgery residency education and training over the last decade (2009–2019). Neurosurg Focus 2020;48(3):E6.

61. Scallon S, Fairholm D, Cochrane D, et al. Evaluation of the operating room as a surgical teaching venue. Canadian Journal of Surgery Journal Canadien de Chirurgie 1992;35(2):173–6.

62. Waseem T, Baig HM, Yasmeen R, et al. Enriching operating room based student learning experience: exploration of factors and development of curricular guidelines. BMC Med Educ 2022;22(1): 739.

63. Information from the ACGME. Society of Neurological Surgeons. Available at: https://www.societyns. org/resident-education/information-from-the-acgme. Accessed February 6, 2024.

64. McPheeters MJ, Talcott RD, Hubbard ME, et al. Assessing the accuracy of neurological surgery resident case logs at a single institution. Surg Neurol Int 2017;8.

65. Collins C, Dudas L, Johnson M, et al. ACGME operative case log accuracy varies among surgical programs. J Surg Educ 2020;77(6):e78–85.

66. Cadieux M, Healy M, Petrusa E, et al. Implementation of competence by design in Canadian neurosurgery residency programs. Med Teach 2022;44(4): 380–7.

67. Frank JR, Snell L, Englander R, et al. Implementing competency-based medical education: Moving forward. Med Teach 2017;39(6):568–73.

68. Crawford L, Cofie N, Mcewen L, et al. Perceptions and barriers to competency-based education in Canadian postgraduate medical education. J Eval Clin Pract 2020;26(4):1124–31.

69. Choe MS, Huffman LC, Feldman HM, et al. Academic Half-Day Education Experience in Postgraduate Medical Training: A Scoping Review of

Characteristics and Learner Outcomes. Front Med 2022;9:835045.

70. Randall MH, Schreiner AD, Clyburn EB, et al. Effects of an academic half day in a residency program on perceived educational value, resident satisfaction and wellness. Am J Med Sci 2020;360(4):342–7.

71. Liang KE, Bernstein I, Kato Y, et al. Enhancing neurosurgical education in low-and middle-income countries: current methods and new advances. Neurol Med -Chir 2016;56(11):709–15.

72. Benassi P, MacGillivray L, Silver I, et al. The role of morbidity and mortality rounds in medical education: a scoping review. Med Educ 2017;51(5):469–79.

73. Kashiwazaki D, Saito H, Uchino H, et al. Morbidity and mortality conference can reduce avoidable morbidity in neurosurgery: its educational effect on residents and surgical safety outcomes. World Neurosurgery 2020;133:e348–55.

74. Clarke MJ, Frimannsdottir K. Assessment of neurosurgical resident milestone evaluation reporting and feedback processes. Neurosurg Focus 2022; 53(2):E5.

75. Seetharaman R. Pros and Cons: Global Adoption of Competency-Based Medical Education. Acad Med 2023;98(12):1346.

76. Weiss HK, Garcia RM, Omiye JA, et al. A systematic review of neurosurgical care in low-income countries. World neurosurgery: X 2020;5:100068.

77. Perez-Chadid DA, Veiga Silva AC, Asfaw ZK, et al. Needs, Roles, and Challenges of Young Latin American and Caribbean Neurosurgeons. World Neurosurg 2023;176:e190–9.

78. Sader E, Yee P, Hodaie M. Assessing barriers to neurosurgical care in sub-Saharan Africa: the role of resources and infrastructure. World Neurosurgery 2017;98:682–8. e683.

Continuing Education for Global Neurosurgery Graduates
Visiting Surgeons, Skills Teaching, Bootcamps, and Twinning Programs

Julie Woodfield, PhD, FRCS, MSc, MBChB, BSc[a,b,c],*, Jared Reese, MD[d], Roger Hartl, MD[c,e], Jack Rock, MD[d]

KEYWORDS

• Global neurosurgery • Education • Bootcamps • Teaching

KEY POINTS

• Postgraduate neurosurgery training programs globally may lack in depth exposure to the breadth of techniques, conditions, or training methods.
• Collaborations with visiting surgeons, bootcamps, skills teaching, or twinning programs can aid in addressing postgraduate training needs.
• For maximum impact and best use of resources, the content and methods of international support need to be identified by the recipients.
• Long-term relationships and "train the trainers" approaches may be more impactful than short-term relationships.

INTRODUCTION

Postgraduate training in neurosurgery in regions such as North America, Europe, and Australasia is delivered through established residency programs. These usually involve immersive supervised experience in patient management and decision-making, practical and surgical skills teaching with hands-on experience, theoretical teaching, and self-directed learning.[1–5] Training is delivered not only from experienced neurosurgeons, but also from interdisciplinary team members and allied specialties such as neuroradiology, neuroanaesthesia and critical care, neurology, and neuropathology. However, in regions where neurosurgery is in the process of becoming established and there are relatively few neurosurgeons, institutional knowledge and experience, support of experts from allied specialties, and support from educationalists for designing and delivering comprehensive competency based neurosurgical postgraduate education may be lacking.[6] When this is compounded with difficulties in access to equipment, literature, online resources, funding, technical support, or even more basic necessities such as a constant clean water and electricity supply, it is not surprising that there is a gap in the available and accessible postgraduate training in neurosurgery between low and high income countries.

a Centre for Clinical Brain Sciences, University of Edinburgh, Edinburgh, UK; b Muhimbili Orthopaedic Institute, Dar es Salaam, Tanzania; c Weill Cornell Medicine Center for Comprehensive Spine Care, 240 E 59th Street, 2nd Floor, New York, NY 10022, USA; d Henry Ford Health, Department of Neurosurgery, 2799 W Grand Boulevard, K11, Detroit, MI 48202, USA; e Och Spine, New York Presbyterian Hospital, New York, USA
* Corresponding author. Department of Clinical Neurosciences, 50 Little France Crescent, Edinburgh, EH16 4TJ, UK.
E-mail address: julie.woodfield@ed.ac.uk

Neurosurg Clin N Am 35 (2024) 439–448
https://doi.org/10.1016/j.nec.2024.05.006
1042-3680/24/© 2024 Elsevier Inc. All rights are reserved, including those for text and data mining, AI training, and similar technologies.

Postgraduate neurosurgery training and fellowships continue to evolve to create neurosurgeons equipped to serve the changing needs and expectations of their populations.[3–5] This necessarily means that different countries and regions have different methods of training, standard setting, and assessment along with differences in practice and health care settings.[2,4] However, efforts have been made in cross-border standardization of common aspects of curriculums and assessment. For example, the European Board examination in Neurological Surgery, and the Fellow of the College of Surgeons in Neurosurgery examination of the College of Surgeons of East, Central and Southern Africa have been introduced along with curricula that span numerous countries within their regions.[2,4,7] Recognizing the common generic aspects of neurosurgery allows neurosurgical knowledge and experience sharing on a global scale. However, the current reality for many neurosurgeons in low or middle income countries is difficulty in accessing training delivered either locally or abroad.[8]

We present here some methods in which global partnerships can work to improve access to post graduate training in neurosurgery where gaps in training exist. We describe our experience of visiting surgeons, team trips, surgical skills teaching, bootcamps, and twinning programs. We concentrate on 2 examples of global partnerships. The first is between the Henry Ford Hospital, Detroit, USA and the Department of Neurosurgery in Yangon and North Okkalappa General Hospital, both in Myanmar. The second is between Weill Cornell Medicine, New York, USA and the Muhimbili Orthopedic Institute, Dar es Salaam, Tanzania. We describe how short and medium term support can strengthen, develop, and empower local and regional postgraduate training systems. Training neurosurgeons to deliver excellent care, defined within their cultural and health care settings, develop world-leading techniques, and to become global centers of excellence in training future generations is the overall goal of these partnerships.[6]

VISITING SURGEONS AND TEAMS

Many collaborations develop from surgeons taking short trips between departments in the hope of learning from each other. Visits lasting between 1 week and 1 month provide the opportunity to get to know one another and understand each other's needs. For example, the programme between the Department of Neurosurgery at Henry Ford Hospital, Detroit, USA and the Department of Neurosurgery in Yangon, Myanmar under the auspices of the Foundation for International Education in Neurosurgery (FIENS) began with 2 years of short single surgeon visits to Dr Win Myaing and Dr Kyi Hlaing in Yangon by Dr Jack Rock from Henry Ford Hospital.[9] This time was spent giving teaching sessions and undertaking joint operating, as well as sharing leisure time. The advantages of single surgeon short trips include the opportunity to spend time getting to know colleagues with different experiences and backgrounds, and identifying shared goals.

Working side-by-side intra-operatively is one frequent benefit and reason for undertaking short trips. Both the visitor and the host surgeon have the opportunity to learn from each other, and patients can benefit from expertise not usually available to them. However, there is a delicate balance to be struck between the visitor and host, both of whom are frequently excellent surgeons in their own right and experts in their local society and institution. Surgeons from high income countries may be used to working with advanced technology and equipment and need to adapt to working without these in some settings. Joint intra-operative working allows hands-on learning and experience and facilitates practical guidance in performing procedures. Observation without supervised performance limits the value of the teaching and knowledge sharing as it does not train the learner to be surgically independent to manage cases. This can be problematic as short-term trips are necessarily limited in scope and help to manage only a small number of patients. Working together rather than observing each other in the operating room is a more effective and fruitful process that can lead to all surgeons developing skills to manage challenging surgical problems after the visit has ended.

After 2 years of single surgeon trips by Dr Jack Rock from Detroit to Yangon, the need for a team trip was identified to address the multidisciplinary needs of neurosurgical patients. The team from Detroit visiting Yangon included surgeons, physicians, nurses, advanced practice providers, and biomedical technicians. Including a range of specialists facilitates addressing the multiple needs of neurosurgical patients during their care pathway and training multiple groups of staff. Biomedical personnel are critical to ensure that equipment works smoothly in operating rooms and on the patient floors, particularly if that equipment has been brought with the visitors and is unfamiliar to the hosts. Visiting technicians can also upskill local biomedical engineers on donated, loan, or permanent equipment belonging to the hospital. Team trips ideally serve the hosts in a broader manner than single surgeon visits by providing an environment for joint bidirectional learning for surgeons, residents, nurses, anaesthesiologists, intensive care unit staff, and other allied health care professionals.

Scoliosis team trips to the Muhimbili Orthopedic Institute in Dar es Salaam, Tanzania is another example of repeated short-term team visits. Here the twin goals were providing the clinical service of treatment for scoliosis patients and developing the multidisciplinary expertise needed for a comprehensive scoliosis programme led locally. Team visits to Dar es Salaam between 2020 and 2023 included surgeons from Palestine, Italy, and the USA, as well as a neurophysiologist from Kenya, nurses from the USA, and implant industry representatives from Italy and the USA.[10] The multidisciplinary nature of the trips facilitated comprehensive care and training, including in intra-operative monitoring and equipment and implant care and use. These aspects are essential for a successful scoliosis programme, but difficult to deliver by surgeons working alone. Including team members from different countries can also stimulate discussion and exposure to a variety of techniques and treatment paradigms. However, team trips, like single surgeon trips, suffer from their short-term nature. A drawback of the scoliosis programme is that yearly 1 week periods do not lend themselves to supporting skills development and consolidation over time as would be the case in a year-long fellowship in a specialist area such as scoliosis surgery. Online learning and support meetings before and after the trips can help address this, as described for the scoliosis training programme.[11]

SKILLS TEACHING

Learning neurosurgical skills requires both theoretical and practical hands-on knowledge. The global neurosurgery course held at the Muhimbili Orthopedic Institute in Dar es Salaam, Tanzania in partnership with Weill Cornell Medicine, New York, USA is one example of a training course tailored to fill a gap in postgraduate neurosurgical education in a low-middle income country (**Fig. 1**). The topics covered by this course are determined by the organizing committee in Tanzania. The course has changed with the development of neurosurgical services in Tanzania over the last 10 years from focusing on neurotrauma and neurocritical care when there were only a handful of neurosurgeons, limited neurointensive care provision, and the service focused on trauma provision.[12] In 2023, there were over 20 neurosurgeons in Tanzania, and the course covered all subspecialties of neurosurgery including vascular, epilepsy, and skull base.[13] This shows how training

courses develop with the needs of the participants. Prior to the course, self-rating of knowledge and confidence in these newer topics, such as neurovascular surgery were lower than the established topics such as trauma, but attendees reported increases in knowledge in all topics following the course.[13,14] Teaching on training, research, and quality improvement was also delivered in the last 2 years, with the recognition that training the trainers of tomorrow and continuous improvement in outcomes are essential for a sustainable service and training programme.[13,14] In line with this, over the last decade, this course has shifted from the majority of faculty visiting from the USA to faculty from Tanzania and other East African nations.[13] Formal and informal feedback from participants and organisers is used to identify teaching methods and topics needed, which is essential to ensure the course develops to address current training needs.[13,14] Recognition of the training course for continuous professional development by both the Medical Council of Tanganyika and the Tanzania Nursing and Midwifery Council ensures regulatory approval and formal recognition of training for participants within regulatory systems.[13,14]

Intra-operative skills teaching as part of the 2023 Dar es Salaam Global Neurosurgery course and previous years included hands-on training in the operating room with both visiting surgeons and local surgeons, as well as training from industry representatives.[13] To maximise learning, cases were presented for discussion in advance, teaching continued throughout the cases, and a review of the experience was presented afterward for discussion. Hands-on surgical training was rated highly by participants.[13] However, it was found that careful case selection was essential for intra-operative training. Visiting surgeons can be at risk of forgetting that the support systems of neuroanaesthesia, critical care, neurosurgical nursing, pharmacy services, and neuroradiology are different than in their home countries. Expecting the same outcomes as in a high income country, or underestimating the local setting can potentially lead to patient harm. Appropriate risk management and careful working with a good listening relationship between all partners can mitigate but not eliminate patient risk. Further, recognition that the appropriateness of surgical intervention or non-intervention, or type of procedure can depend on diagnostic and adjuvant treatments available is essential for ethical decision making, particularly in the area of neuro-oncology where neuropathologic diagnosis may be limited to histology and chemo-radiotherapy inaccessible in many settings.

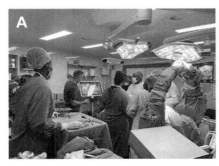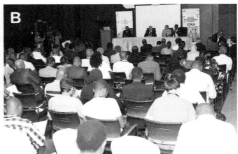

Fig. 1. The Dar es Salaam Global Neurosurgery Course 2023. (*A*) Intraoperative learning with Brainlab for spinal fixation (*B*) Neurotrauma question and answer session.

Simulation training in neurosurgery is low risk to patients and there is evidence that it improves knowledge and technical skills.[15] After attending a course using Upsurgeon[16] cranial approaches simulators in Nairobi, Kenya, organized prior to the Congress of Continental Association of African Neurosurgeons in 2022, Tanzanian neurosurgeons worked in conjunction with Weill Cornell Medicine, New York, to add simulation training to the Global Neurosurgery Course in Dar es Salaam, Tanzania in 2023. The Upsurgeon simulators combine high fidelity cranial approaches in a box with augmented reality, and are low cost, particularly compared to the infrastructure required for cadaveric skills and anatomy teaching, but still have rental and shipping costs.[16] After using the pterional, temporal, retrosigmoid, aneurysm, and tumor simulators, feedback from the simulation course was mostly very positive with attendees finding the simulation easy and intuitive to use and stating the sessions would improve their surgical practice (**Fig. 2**),[13] similar to another Upsurgeon simulation course held in Cameroon.[17] Further evidence of the perceived benefit was the request of the residents to continue the simulation teaching sessions weekly. However, use of the augmented reality feature required access to a smartphone supporting this and many smartphones in use in the region were incompatible.[13] Downloading of the applications to support the teaching also required a smartphone and good internet access. These were surmountable challenges with sharing of devices and internet connectivity, but technological challenges such as these need consideration and robust plans for management or alternatives in the event of failure. Attempts at virtual reality pedicle screw insertion simulation encountered similar connectivity and infrastructure challenges, but the training was felt to be beneficial.[13] Feedback from previous Real Spine lumbar spine surgical simulation training was similarly positive,[18] showing that both cranial and spinal approaches

can be successfully taught using simulation around the world.

BOOTCAMPS

Bootcamps were introduced by the Society of Neurological Surgeons in 2010 as regional training courses for first year neurosurgery residents in the USA covering core fundamental skills, knowledge, and attitudes.[19] This was in response to a change in training responsibility whereby the first postgraduate year of training was incorporated into neurosurgery residency training and the recognition that core skills and knowledge training could be delivered in a standard format regionally or nationally.[19] The model of a 2 day training course on the basics of neurosurgical care and experience in procedures that will be performed during residency has worked well, with good knowledge retention on follow-up.[20] The bootcamp model is based on standardised training of a specified curriculum with stated aims. This model of basic skills training in neurosurgery has since been adopted in many other countries. In the United Kingdom, residents now attend 1 week bootcamps in year 1 of neurosurgery training on basic knowledge, skills, and procedures, in year 3 on more advanced operative techniques, and in year 8 on leadership and management. Bootcamps with standardised curricula aimed at neurosurgery residents provide a model for training in fundamental aspects of knowledge, skills, and attitudes, and reports of the impact of bootcamps from Myanmar, Bolivia, Vietnam, South Africa, and Pakistan in improving skills have been positive.[9,21,22]

The preparation required to execute a successful bootcamp cannot be underestimated.[9] Preparatory work for the international faculty can take 4 to 6 months. For simulation or practical activities, communication, and involvement of industry sponsors that are willing to support a bootcamp also play a critical role. Company connections

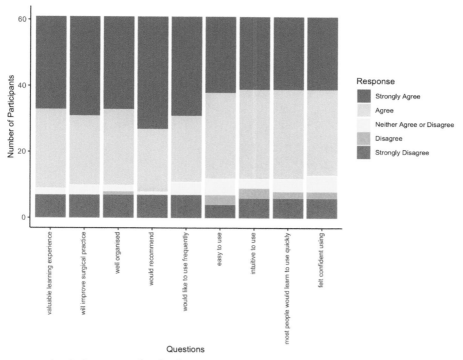

Fig. 2. Upsurgeon simulation course feedback. 60 participants were asked for feedback about the Upsurgeon simulation course held in Dar es Salaam in March 2023 and the graph represents the responses from the feedback questionnaire.

can provide access and transportation of equipment so that trainees are exposed to basic neurosurgical procedures and, additionally, the company representatives can assist with training at workstations. Successful teaching of key information requires clearly defined roles and responsibilities for each activity for those involved, and learning can be multi-modality, including preparatory online lectures, in-person didactic teaching, small group case-based discussions, and hands-on workstations.

In 2017, the first South East Asia Yangon neurosurgery bootcamp was held with the support of Medtronic, Storz and Integra,[9] and bootcamps have continued in Singapore (2018), Yangon (2019), and Danang (2022). Generally, these bootcamps host 40 to 50 neurosurgery residents and 15 to 25 faculty members, both local and international. The first day of the Yangon bootcamp in 2017 (shown in **Fig. 3**) included didactic teaching on the management of patients with a traumatic brain injury, hydrocephalus, spinal cord compression, stroke, subarachnoid haemorrhage, intracerebral haemorrhage, pituitary lesions, and common surgical approaches such as anterior and posterior cervical fusions, and surgical techniques for the treatment of brain tumors.[9]

Breakout sessions for small group case-based discussions were focused on common neurosurgical emergencies.[9] On the second day of the bootcamp, hands-on workstations included cranial positioning, lumbar punctures, shunt taps, intracranial pressure monitor and external ventricular drain placement, endoscopic transnasal approaches, lumbar pedicle screw placement, and cranial work (including craniotomy drilling, microscope use, dural closure, plating, and skin closure).[9] Each workstation was provided with a checklist of steps to perform during each procedure. All bootcamp participants worked with experienced faculty, both locally and internationally, rendering a unique teaching environment for them to actively participate in.[9]

The benefits of the bootcamp model of standardised training against set curricula are that the bootcamp contents and curriculum can be planned to address local needs, the standardised curricula facilitate repetition in future years, and the explicitly stated objectives aid in training and empowerment of faculty to teach, gain experience in developing curricula, and pass on skills. For this to be successful, it is imperative that the training needs and background of the residents are adequately taken into consideration, as well as

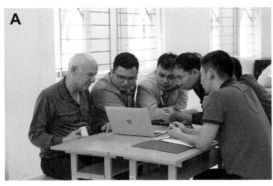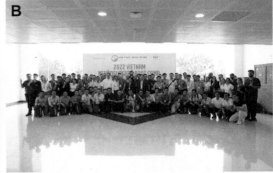

Fig. 3. The Danang Bootcamp 2022 (*A*) Participants reviewing cases with Dr Russell Andrews (*B*) All participants at the Danang Bootcamp in December 2022.

the equipment available and environment in which usual practice occurs. For example, if usual practice is using a Hudson brace to perform burr holes then training with an electric perforator will not facilitate everyday care. Bootcamps have the potential to improve patient care in both young and old neurosurgery training programmes through standardised training of core skills, but must also develop over time to stay relevant to the needs of those attending.

NEUROSURGICAL TWINNING PROGRAMMES

The approach of twinning programmes between neurosurgical departments across the world addresses the issues of short-term or one-off post graduate neurosurgical education methods. Twinning programmes involve a medium or long-term commitment to joint development and learning. A formal arrangement and commitment can facilitate long-term widespread development in training, research, facilities, and leadership.

In 2015, after 4 years of working together, a formal twinning programme was established between the Yangon General Hospital in Myanmar and the Henry Ford Hospital, Detroit, USA. Formalities included a signed Memorandum of Understanding and approval from the Ministry of Health in Myanmar. Governmental support, particularly of government-run hospitals, can be essential to facilitate development of a national neurosurgery training programme, placement of trained neurosurgeons in regional hospitals and organisation of services, and expanding provision of facilities required for patient care. The twinning programme between Yangon and Detroit has led to the development of a formal training programme curriculum for residency in Yangon, yearly visits of staff from the Henry Ford Hospital to Yangon to teach both nurses and residents, 6 to 8 week observerships at the Henry Ford's Department of Neurosurgery

for Yangon residents, and the development of the bootcamps described above.[9]

In 2018, the Henry Ford Hospital in Detroit, USA twinned with the North Okkalappa General Hospital, Myanmar, where team trips continued with neurosurgery residents from the Henry Ford joining the team, and the beginning of bi-weekly online educational meetings between residents in Myanmar and Detroit to discuss important topics in neurosurgery and patient care. In 2019, this culminated in an award from the Congress of Neurologic Surgeons for work on traumatic brain injury. Since 2016, the twinning programme has also worked to get educational grants from medical instrument and equipment companies in support of equipment needs for a number of surgical procedures including cranial nerve monitors (Medtronic), endoscopes (Storz), aneurysm clips (SurgicalOne and Mizuho) and others, depending on the needs of the departments in Yangon and North Okkalappa. The long-term twinning programme facilitates an environment in which needed equipment can be procured, sustainably serviced, and trained with. This avoids the hazards of equipment donations outside of a twinning programme where there are risks of unwanted, un-needed, unusable or inappropriate equipment being sourced that may not be useful.

As of January 2020, in conjunction with the FIENS and at the request of Dr. Myaing and Hlaing in Myanmar, a written neurosurgical academic curriculum was developed and the faculty and residents at the North Okkalappa General Hospital began meeting weekly to present and discuss important and diverse topics prepared in advance by the faculty and residents. The neurosurgery residents in Myanmar have played a critical role in all of the activities and academic work of the twinning programme, and will continue to be involved going forward. Unfortunately, since the coup in February 2021, the twinning programme between the Henry Ford Hospital and the North Okkalappa General Hospital has not been able to proceed, but hopefully will be reestablished in the future. Political and governmental stability and support is necessary for a successful twinning programme.

A longstanding neurosurgical twinning programme also exists between the Muhumbili Orthopedic Institute in Dar es Salaam, Tanzania and the Weill Cornell Medicine in New York, USA. This has grown over the past 10 years to include a yearly neurosurgery training course in Dar es Salaam,[12,14] cost-free 3 month observerships in New York for Tanzanian neurosurgeons, residents, and nurses, a junior research fellowship in Dar es Salaam, and a year-long fellowship for a Western trained neurosurgeon to work in Tanzania to support the programme. Weekly online meetings, plus collaborative clinical and research projects in traumatic spine injury, traumatic brain injury, epilepsy, and other topics provide training and experience in clinical care, service improvement, operative skills and research. Equipment donations, such as a recently donated Brainlab machine from the RightBrain Foundation are supported by this twinning programme to ensure training, maintenance, access to consumables, and continued support for its use.[13] **Box 1** shows possible components of global neurosurgery twinning programmes.

In addition to supporting neurosurgeons directly, the twinning programme between the Muhimbili Orthopedic Institute and the Weill Cornell Medicine has broadened the support for safe neurosurgical care by training staff in intraoperative monitoring through hands-on training both in New York and visiting neurophysiologists in Tanzania, and supporting the neuroscience nursing education programme-training and empowering nurses to deliver training both at the Muhimbili Orthopedic Institute and across Tanzania. Institutional twinning programmes have the advantage of a multidisciplinary approach, upskilling many professionals involved in neurosurgical care and offsetting problems encountered where surgical skills develop

without institutional multidisciplinary support for safe and effective care.

Long-term twinning programmes can also facilitate a culture of lifelong joint learning with assessment of local outcomes and adjustment of techniques and protocols to continuously improve care and outcomes. One-off teaching without this has the danger of introducing concepts and techniques that become disproven or replaced, or can cause inadvertent harm in the setting. For example, a quicker time to surgery for cervical spine injuries was associated with increased mortality in Dar es Salaam, leading to emphasis on resuscitation and medical care first rather than speed to spinal fixation. This highlights how the sharing of skills in critical appraisal, data evaluation, research, and quality improvement is just as important if not more important than sharing of current surgical skills. The structure of a twinning programme can help provide a scaffold on which short-term visits and equipment, teaching, and data analysis can have maximum impact.

DISCUSSION

It is estimated that more than 23,000 additional neurosurgeons are required worldwide to provide neurosurgical care for the population,[23] and the majority of these are needed in South East Asia and Africa[23]—the same regions where gaps in provision of neurosurgical training exist.[7,8,24–27] Self-sustaining high quality neurosurgical training programmes available and accessible to local doctors are essential to deliver safe affordable surgical care whilst continuously improving standards and training the next generation of neurosurgeons.[28] Although international support through visiting surgeons, training courses, and twinning programmes can have a valuable impact on training and care provision, all of these must work toward strengthening the local and regional training systems to provide high quality self-sustaining in-country training and service.[28]

Challenges for postgraduate education in neurosurgery globally include balancing the provision of time and resources for teaching with service needs, training of neurosurgeons in teaching methodology, engagement of other specialties in neurosurgical education, and a structure for ensuring breadth and depth of access to subspecialty training, particularly where conditions are uncommon.[3–5,24,27,29,30] Costs for training are another barrier, and these may be amplified in low or middle income countries and systems where residents pay training fees and may not receive a salary.[27,29,31] Some of these challenges can be helped through international collaboration

---

Box 1
Components of global neurosurgery twinning programmes

- Short-term visits between departments
- Training courses
- Fellowships/observerships for multidisciplinary team members in both departments
- Joint research projects and publications
- Regular online meetings

bringing free courses, skills teaching, and visits.[24,32] However, it must be emphasized that the usefulness of these initiatives relies on proactively identifying needs, appropriate teaching methods and content.

Historically in global medicine and neurosurgery, knowledge flows have been from high income to low and middle income settings. However, in a truly global setting, learning is multi-directional. For example, the cure hydrocephalus programme in Uganda has trained many neurosurgeons from both high and low income countries in neuro-endoscopy,[33] and both Cape Town, South Africa, and Rabat, Morrocco regularly train neurosurgeons from other African countries.[28,34,35] The benefits of training in a setting similar to that in which you will be providing care with those whose regular practice mirrors yours, and training with patients who present similarly to those you expect to treat are inestimable.[33] Neurosurgical trainers aim for their trainees to surpass them in knowledge and skills, and the ultimate aim of global collaboration should be for a rounded neurosurgical community in which local training is delivered by trained knowledgeable trainers locally, and then subspecialist or fellowship training offered on a global scale in conditions and techniques with expertise in that region, for example, in hydrocephalus in Mbale, Uganda,[33] low grade glioma management in Montpellier, France,[36] and neurovascular training in Helsinki, Finland.[37]

By the inherent nature of this planned special journal issue and invited authorship, this article is limited by its views of those looking at global neurosurgery from a background in high income countries. Although there are some general principles of training initiatives, it has been shown many times that working to local priorities and needs determines maximum impact.[28] Gains for those from high income countries from participating in training in a global settting cannot be underestimated, with access to training and teaching experience and conditions that may be rare in high income countries.[38] In all endeavors, the flow of resource from low to high income countries, making an already inequitable situation less equitable should be avoided. This balance is particularly difficult where funding for initiatives in low income countries flows to high income institutions, strengthening their resources rather than supporting infrastructure and development of skills, facilities, and human resources in the under-resourced setting. Another limitation of this article is that many of the experiences described are not critically evaluated for their long-term impact, or their impact on other areas of the health care system. Training neurosurgeons has been shown to improve trauma, surgical and anaesthetics care across the health service,[39,40] but there is also the risk of causing harm socio-culturally or to systems through development of a single service, and the wider impact of initiatives should be carefully studied.[41] Recognition that each country and each learner is an individual and there is no one size fits all best case solution for either training or neurosurgical practice is essential to working together on a global scale to improve training and patient care worldwide.

SUMMARY

There is currently a gap between postgraduate neurosurgery training available around the world. We have presented some methods by which departments, surgeons, and teams can contribute to closing that gap, with the aim of establishing a circular global neurosurgery economy where individual countries and regions recognize their own needs and strengths and share those strengths with other departments whilst receiving assistance with needs.

CLINICS CARE POINTS

- Global neurosurgical collaborations aiming to improve postgraduate training have included methods such as visiting surgeons and teams, bootcamps, skills teaching, and twinning programmes.

- Bootcamps and skills training deliver training in specific generic neurosurgical skills appropriate to the setting, and can be developed and led by local faculty for maximum impact.

- Twinning programmes have the advantage of capacity strengthening to address long-term goals, involvement and training of multidisciplinary teams, and ability to support infrastructure and equipment.

- The overall aim of global collaboration in training methods is to support development of self-sustaining relevant training appropriate to the needs of the participants.

DISCLOSURE

R. Hartl declares consulting work for DePuy Synthes and Brainlab. R. Hartl reports a financial relationship with Zimmer Biomet and Realist. No other author declares any financial interests or personal relationships.

REFERENCES

1. Sealy WC. Halsted is dead: Time for change in graduate surgical education. Curr Surg 1999;56(1):34–9.
2. Grotenhuis A, Świątkowska-Wróblewska K, Sala F, et al. Neurosurgery education around the world: Europe. In: Germano IM, editor. Neurosurgery and global health. Springer International Publishing; 2022. p. 229–38.
3. Selden NR, Barbaro NM, Barrow DL, et al. Neurosurgery residency and fellowship education in the United States: 2 decades of system development by the One Neurosurgery Summit organizations. J Neurosurg 2022;136(2):565–74.
4. Whitfield PC, Van Loon J, Peul W, Executive Board of the European Association of Neurosurgical S. European training requirements in neurological surgery: A new outcomes-based 3 stage UEMS curriculum. Brain Spine 2023;3:101744.
5. Morgan MK, Clarke RM, Lyon PM, et al. The neurosurgical training curriculum in Australia and New Zealand is changing. Why? J Clin Neurosci 2005; 12(2):115–8.
6. Bankole NDA, Ouahabi AE. Towards a collaborative-integrative model of education and training in neurosurgery in low and middle-income countries. Clin Neurol Neurosurg 2022;220:107376.
7. Mulwafu W, Fualal J, Bekele A, et al. The impact of COSECSA in developing the surgical workforce in East Central and Southern Africa. Surgeon 2022; 20(1):2–8.
8. Deora H, Garg K, Tripathi M, et al. Residency perception survey among neurosurgery residents in lower-middle-income countries: grassroots evaluation of neurosurgery education. Neurosurg Focus 2020;48(3):E11.
9. Rock J, Glick R, Germano IM, et al. The first neurosurgery boot camp in southeast asia: evaluating impact on knowledge and regional collaboration in Yangon, Myanmar. World Neurosurg 2018;113:e239–46.
10. Waterkeyn F, Ikwuegbuenyi CA, Woodfield J, et al. Evaluating the feasibility and outcomes of a scoliosis surgical camp in a resource-limited setting in sub-saharan Africa. World Neurosurg 2023;180:e550–9.
11. Ahmad AA, Abushehab A, Waterkeyn F, et al. The efficacy of blended learning in a pediatric spine deformity management program in sub-Saharan Africa. J Am Acad Orthop Surg Glob Res Rev 2023;7(2).
12. Kahamba JF, Assey AB, Dempsey RJ, et al. The second African Federation of Neurological Surgeons course in the East, Central, and Southern Africa region held in Dar es Salaam, Tanzania, January 2011. World Neurosurg 2013;80(3–4):255–9.
13. Shayo CS, Woodfield J, Shabhay ZA, et al. Neurosurgical Education in Tanzania: The Dar es Salaam Global Neurosurgery Course. World Neurosurg 2023;180:42–51.
14. Waterkeyn F, Woodfield J, Massawe SL, et al. The effect of the Dar es Salaam neurosurgery training course on self-reported neurosurgical knowledge and confidence. Brain and Spine 2023;3:101727.
15. Davids J, Manivannan S, Darzi A, et al. Simulation for skills training in neurosurgery: a systematic review, meta-analysis, and analysis of progressive scholarly acceptance. Neurosurg Rev 2021;44(4):1853–67.
16. Petrone S, Cofano F, Nicolosi F, et al. Virtual-Augmented Reality and Life-Like Neurosurgical Simulator for Training: First Evaluation of a Hands-On Experience for Residents. Front Surg 2022;9: 862948.
17. Takoutsing BD, Wunde UN, Zolo Y, et al. Assessing the impact of neurosurgery and neuroanatomy simulation using 3D non-cadaveric models amongst selected African medical students. Front Med Technol 2023;5:1190096.
18. Balogun SA, Sommer F, Waterkeyn F, et al. Feasibility of High-Fidelity Simulator Models for Minimally Invasive Spine Surgery in a Resource-Limited Setting: Experience From East Africa. J Am Acad Orthop Surg Glob Res Rev 2023;7(10).
19. Selden NR, Origitano TC, Burchiel KJ, et al. A national fundamentals curriculum for neurosurgery PGY1 residents: the 2010 Society of Neurological Surgeons boot camp courses. Neurosurgery 2012; 70(4):971–81 [discussion 981].
20. Selden NR, Anderson VC, McCartney S, et al. Society of Neurological Surgeons boot camp courses: knowledge retention and relevance of hands-on learning after 6 months of postgraduate year 1 training. J Neurosurg 2013;119(3):796–802.
21. Ament JD, Kim T, Gold-Markel J, et al. Planning and Executing the Neurosurgery Boot Camp: The Bolivia Experience. World Neurosurg 2017;104:407–10.
22. Bakhshi SK, Ahmad R, Merchant AAH, et al. Development, outcome and costs of a simulation-based neurosurgery bootcamp at the national level. BMC Med Educ 2022;22(1):896.
23. Dewan MC, Rattani A, Fieggen G, et al. Global neurosurgery: the current capacity and deficit in the provision of essential neurosurgical care. Executive Summary of the Global Neurosurgery Initiative at the Program in Global Surgery and Social Change. J Neurosurg 2018;1–10.
24. Ferraris KP, Matsumura H, Wardhana DPW, et al. The state of neurosurgical training and education in East Asia: analysis and strategy development for this frontier of the world. Neurosurg Focus 2020;48(3):E7.
25. Beer-Furlan A, Neto SG, Teixeira MJ, et al. Fulfilling Need for Neurosurgical Services in Sub-Saharan Africa: Initial Angola-Brazil Training Experience. World Neurosurg 2019;122:29–32.
26. Dada OE, Karekezi C, Mbangtang CB, et al. State of Neurosurgical Education in Africa: A Narrative Review. World Neurosurg 2021;151:172–81.

27. Elmaraghi S, Park KM, Rashidian N, et al. Postgraduate Surgical Education in East, Central, and Southern Africa: A Needs Assessment Survey. J Am Coll Surg 2022. https://doi.org/10.1097/XCS.000000000 0000457.

28. Dempsey RJ, Buckley NA. Education-based Solutions to the Global Burden of Neurosurgical Disease. World Neurosurg 2020;140:e1–6.

29. Sader E, Yee P, Hodaie M. Barriers to Neurosurgical Training in Sub-Saharan Africa: The Need for a Phased Approach to Global Surgery Efforts to Improve Neurosurgical Care. World Neurosurg 2017;98:397–402.

30. Henderson F Jr, Abdifatah K, Qureshi M, et al. The College of Surgeons of East, Central, and Southern Africa: Successes and Challenges in Standardizing Neurosurgical Training. World Neurosurg 2020;136: 172–7.

31. Kanmounye US, Zolo Y, Tsopmene MRD, et al. Understanding the motivations, needs, and challenges faced by aspiring neurosurgeons in Africa: an E-survey. Br J Neurosurg 2022;36(1):38–43.

32. Onyia CU, Ojo OA. Collaborative International Neurosurgery Education for Africa-The Journey So Far and the Way Forward. World Neurosurg 2020; 141:e566–75.

33. Warf BC. Educate one to save a few. Educate a few to save many. World Neurosurg 2013;79(2 Suppl): S15.e15–8.

34. Karekezi C, El Khamlichi A. Takeoff of African Neurosurgery and the World Federation of Neurosurgical

35. Karekezi C, El Khamlichi A, El Ouahabi A, et al. The impact of African-trained neurosurgeons on sub-Saharan Africa. Neurosurg Focus 2020;48(3):E4.

36. Duffau H, Taillandier L. New concepts in the management of diffuse low-grade glioma: Proposal of a multistage and individualized therapeutic approach. Neuro Oncol 2015;17(3):332–42.

37. Lehecka ML A, Hernesniemi J. Helsinki microneurosurgery basics and tricks. 1st edition. Helsinki: Druckerei Hohl GmbH & Co; 2011.

38. Gandy K, Castillo H, Rocque BG, et al. Neurosurgical training and global health education: systematic review of challenges and benefits of in-country programs in the care of neural tube defects. Neurosurg Focus 2020;48(3):E14.

39. Haglund MM, Kiryabwire J, Parker S, et al. Surgical capacity building in Uganda through twinning, technology, and training camps. World J Surg 2011; 35(6):1175–82.

40. Haglund MM, Warf B, Fuller A, et al. Past, Present, and Future of Neurosurgery in Uganda. Neurosurgery 2017;80(4):656–61.

41. Lu Z, Tshimbombu TN, Abu-Bonsrah N, et al. Transnational capacity building efforts in global neurosurgery: a review and analysis of their impact and determinants of success. World Neurosurg 2023; 173:188–98.e3.

Societies Rabat Training Center Alumni. World Neurosurg 2019;126:576–80.

Establishing Microsurgery Skills Laboratories in Low- and Middle-income Countries with Integrated Remote Teaching: A Novel Approach

Abdullah Keles, MD[a], Garret P. Greeneway, MD[a], Robert J. Dempsey, MD[a], Mustafa K. Baskaya, MD[a],*

KEYWORDS

- Bypass curriculum • Global neurosurgery • Laboratory training • LMIC • Microanastomosis
- Microsurgery • Remote teaching • Self-assessment

KEY POINTS

- Starting in the late 1960s, neurosurgery has undergone significant advancements with the introduction of microsurgical techniques.
- Owing to limited infrastructure, equipment, and training opportunities, low- and middle-income countries (LMICs) have struggled to fully benefit from these advanced microsurgical techniques.
- We established Madison Microneurosurgery Initiative to address disparities in microsurgery laboratory training for health care professionals from LMICs in their home countries.
- Our novel approach of combining microsurgery training kits with live-streamed training sessions and Madison Objective Self-Assessment Tool has made remote microsurgery laboratory training feasible in LMICs.

INTRODUCTION

In the late 1960s, neurosurgery experienced a significant advancement with the introduction of microsurgery, following the groundbreaking laboratory research conducted by leading neurosurgeons.[1,2] Despite these microsurgical advancements, the distribution of advanced neurosurgical treatments has been uneven globally, resulting in a widening gap between high-income countries (HICs) and low- and middle-income countries (LMICs).[3] This gap in neurosurgical care is mainly due to disparities in infrastructure, availability of advanced equipment, and skilled health care workers, along with a notable lack of microsurgery laboratory training facilities and professionals trained in microsurgical techniques. In those LMICs where advanced treatment options such as endovascular procedures and radiosurgery are inaccessible, the use of microneurosurgical techniques remains crucial for managing neurosurgical diseases.

THE UNIVERSITY OF WISCONSIN–MADISON MICRONEUROSURGERY LABORATORY

The University of Wisconsin–Madison Microneurosurgery Laboratory, directed by one of the authors (MKB), provides a unique platform for worldwide medical professionals, featuring a variety of

[a] Department of Neurological Surgery, University of Wisconsin School of Medicine and Public Health, 600 Highland Avenue, CSC K4/884, Madison, WI 53792, USA
* Corresponding author.
E-mail address: baskaya@neurosurgery.wisc.edu

Neurosurg Clin N Am 35 (2024) 449–463
https://doi.org/10.1016/j.nec.2024.05.007
1042-3680/24/© 2024 Elsevier Inc. All rights reserved, including those for text and data mining, AI training, and similar technologies.

programs: microvascular bypass training, clinical and operating room observership, access to the Microneurosurgery Video Archive of one of the senior authors (MKB), research opportunities, hands-on cadaver dissections, and participation in departmental meetings and annual courses.

From 2006 until the Covid-19 pandemic era in 2020, our laboratory welcomed over 200 international fellows from more than 18 countries across 5 continents.[4] In the period following Covid-19 pandemic, specifically since May 2021, the laboratory has hosted 62 international research fellows and observers from 27 countries. Of these trainees, 90% (56 individuals) came from LMICs, while 10% (6 individuals) were from HICs.

While our laboratory serves as a key facility offering unique opportunity for medical professionals globally, health care workers from LMICs face several challenges in visiting our laboratory to learn and practice advanced microsurgical techniques. These obstacles range from geographic distance and visa requirements to travel and accommodation expenses, currency exchange rates, as well as cultural and linguistic differences.

BASKAYA MICROVASCULAR BYPASS TRAINING CURRICULUM

The initial microneurosurgery laboratory training primarily focused on intracranial arterial thrombectomy and microsuturing techniques, with significant work being conducted in microsurgery laboratories in Burlington, Vermont.[5,6] It was here that Professor Yasargil spent 14 months mastering his microvascular surgery skills, especially in microsuturing.[7] This rigorous training set the stage for notable surgical breakthroughs. Professor Yasargil, after this period of intensive microsurgery training, executed the first successful superficial temporal artery–middle cerebral artery (STA-MCA) bypass procedure on a patient in Zurich. Shortly thereafter, Professor Donaghy achieved the second successful STA-MCA bypass procedure in Burlington the following day.[8] Furthermore, Professor Yasargil applied these refined microsurgery techniques across various neurosurgical domains, skillfully addressing a multitude of pathologies such as arterio-venous malformations (AVMs), aneurysms, and tumors.[9] These advancements underscore the crucial role of microsuturing training. It is not merely a specialized skill; it is a fundamental, versatile combination of techniques applicable in a wide array of neurosurgical procedures.

Since 2006, our laboratory has been offering the Baskaya Microvascular Bypass Training Curriculum (BMBTC) for medical professionals, with its most recent revision and update implemented in 2021 by the first author. It covers fundamental suturing and microvascular anastomosis techniques using a variety of materials and sutures (**Table 1**).

In the first section of the BMBTC, trainees begin by practicing continuous suturing on a Penrose drain, designed to provide foundational skills pertinent to carotid endarterectomy procedures. Furthermore, starting with larger needles, thicker sutures, and larger training materials allows learners to adapt to working under low microscopic magnification (6x - 10x) and to familiarize themselves with the use of microsurgical instruments.

In the second section, the size of the practice materials is reduced from inches to millimeters. Trainees complete multiple attempts at end-to-end, end-to-side, and side-to-side anastomosis using 9-0 sutures. In this section, trainees are introduced to the basic microvascular anastomosis techniques and gain experience with smaller materials and sutures, all under high microscopic magnification (12x - 15x).

In the third section, 10-0 sutures are employed for 3 attempts at each type of anastomosis, utilizing chicken vessels. Chicken vessels serve as ideal biological materials due to their universal availability and lower cost compared to artificial alternatives such as silicone tubes. We usually use chicken thighs as a vessel source, which provides the added benefit of enabling practice in microsurgical dissections under microscopic magnification to locate and expose the vessels.

In the final section, trainees are required to successfully complete at least one anastomosis on live rats under inhalation anesthesia. The femoral artery and veins, carotid arteries, and jugular veins are commonly used for practicing end-to-end and end-to-side anastomosis. For side-to-side anastomosis practice, the inferior vena cava and abdominal aorta are considered ideal.

MADISON OBJECTIVE SELF-ASSESSMENT TOOL

Providing detailed, objective feedback is crucial for effective training in microvascular bypass techniques. We previously developed Madison Objective Self-Assessment Tool (MOST): a specialized self-assessment tool tailored for BMBTC (Madison objective self-assessment tool: a reliable and user-friendly approach for objective self-assessment in microvascular anastomosis training, 2024, unpublished data). MOST not only enables trainees at all levels to independently practice BMBTC and objectively assess the quality of their microsurgical exercises, but it also primarily aims to track and foster continuous improvement in their training. Trainees use MOST metrics to evaluate

Table 1
Baskaya microvascular bypass training curriculum details

Section	Practice Materials	Practice
Section 1	BTK, $1/4$ inch Penrose drain, 6-0 and 7-0 sutures	6 cm continuous suturing practice with Penrose drain; 5 attempts with each suture
Section 2	BTK, 3 and 2 mm silicone tubes, 9-0 suture	E-E, E-S, and S-S anastomosis; 3 attempts E-E anastomosis with 3 mm silicone tubes, 3 attempts E-E anastomosis with 2 mm silicone tubes, 3 attempts E-S anastomosis with 3 mm (recipient) and 2 mm (donor) silicone tubes, and 3 attempts S-S anastomosis with 3 mm silicone tubes
Section 3	BTK, chicken vessel, 10-0 suture	E-E, E-S, and S-S anastomosis; 3 attempts E-E anastomosis, 3 attempts E-S anastomosis, and 3 attempts S-S anastomosis
Section 4	BTK, live rat, 10-0 suture	E-E, E-S, and S-S anastomosis; one successful attempt at one of the anastomosis types

Abbreviations: BTK: basic training kit; E-E, end-to-end; E-S, end-to-side; S-S, side-to-side.

their performance against standard reference scores after completing each of the 31 BMBTC end products (**Table 2**). This helps them identify areas for improvement in future attempts. In LMICs, where expert evaluation can be scarce, MOST proves to be particularly valuable, offering a structured method for trainees to self-assess and enhance their skills.[10]

A NOVEL APPROACH: MADISON MICRONEUROSURGERY INITIATIVE

In February 2020, the Madison Microneurosurgery Initiative (MMI) was established by the first author, at the University of Wisconsin–Madison Microneurosurgery Laboratory. This initiative focuses on addressing existing challenges and closing the gap in microsurgery laboratory training in LMICs. It aims to offer sustainable, accessible, and free microsurgery training solutions to medical professionals in LMICs within their own countries.

ASSEMBLY OF MICROSURGERY TRAINING KITS

To facilitate microsurgery laboratory training in LMICs, initially we expanded our understanding of the requirements for these laboratories. Drawing inspiration from the practices of early microsurgeons and their laboratories, we aimed to recreate their pioneering laboratory setups that were first introduced during the early years of the microsurgery. Additionally, the first author's proficiency in microsurgery laboratories, acquired from foundational experiences at Yeditepe Microneurosurgery Laboratory (Istanbul, Türkiye) and University of Wisconsin–Madison Microneurosurgery Laboratory (Madison, WI, USA), significantly contributed to this work.

Throughout our research period, we evaluated various used stereo microscopes, light sources, and assorted instrument sets, prioritizing cost-effectiveness and quality. This approach led us to uncover pre-owned or surplus stereo microscopes, often sold to the public by university and state surplus departments.

In 2021, after a year of comprehensive research, we established the essential components for microsurgery training kits. Our basic training kit (BTK; **Fig. 1**A) included a stereo microscope with high-quality optics, external light source, a basic set of microsurgery instruments, and practice materials. With additional surgical grade instruments, we set up advanced training kit (ATK; **Fig. 1**B). Subsequently, we began procuring required items from various online auction platforms and additional online sources.

Microscopes

Basic microsurgery training can be effectively conducted using any microscope that ensures enough magnification, high-quality stereoscopic vision, and a suitable working distance. Guided by this knowledge, we explored the use of old tabletop stereo microscopes for microsurgery training. The concept emerged after the first author disassembled, cleaned, and examined an old Zeiss (Jena, West Germany) stereo microscope that had been previously overlooked (**Fig. 2**A, B). Impressed with its optical image quality, we subsequently started looking for similar microscopes on online auction websites.

The initial purchase of a microscope was made on April 26, 2021, for $182. Following this, 4 more microscopes were acquired from the same source, University of Wisconsin–Madison surplus department, at costs of $52, $56, $62, and $70 (**Fig. 2**C).[11]

Table 2
Madison objective self-assessment tool metrics and evaluation criteria

BMBTC Sections	Metrics	Evaluation Criteria
Section 1 Penrose Drain Continuous Suturing Practice	Suture numbers Incision line visuality Suture length Suture interval Needle shape Timing	Number of sutures in 6 cm Edge overlap length in millimeters Number of abnormal sutures (<1 or >2 mm) Number of abnormal intervals (<1 or >2 mm) Normal or distorted Time to complete each attempt
Section 2 Silicone Tube End-to-end, End-to-side, and Side-to-side Anastomosis Practice	Suture numbers (only for E-E) First 4 suture positions (only for E-E and E-S) Back wall continuous suturing Start and end positions (only for S-S) Overlap (only for E-E) Suture interval (only for E-S) Front wall suture interval (only for S-S) Knot quality Back wall gap (only for S-S) Tear Needle shape Timing per suture (only for E-E) Timing (only for E-S and S-S)	Number of sutures to complete anastomosis Number of abnormal suture position Number of sutures causes overlap Number of abnormal intervals (<1 or >2 mm) Number of loose sutures Present or absent Number of tears on the edges Normal or distorted Time to complete each suture (total time/suture number) Time to complete each attempt
Section 3 Chicken Vessel End-to-end, End-to-side, and Side-to-side Anastomosis Practice	Visible sutures Intraluminal tread ends Back wall involvement Back wall gap (only for S-S) Knot quality Needle shape Timing per suture (only for E-E and E-S) Timing (only for S-S)	Ratio of visible sutures in lumen and outside Number of thread ends in the lumen Present or absent Present or absent Number of loose sutures Normal or distorted Time to complete each suture (total time/suture number) Time to complete each attempt

Abbreviations: BMBTC, Baskaya Microvascular Bypass Training Curriculum; E-E, end-to-end; E-S, end-to-side; S-S, side-to-side.

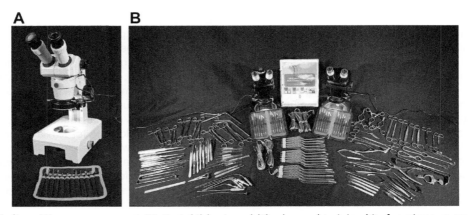

Fig. 1. Madison Microneurosurgery Initiative's (*A*) basic and (*B*) advanced training kits for microsurgery training.

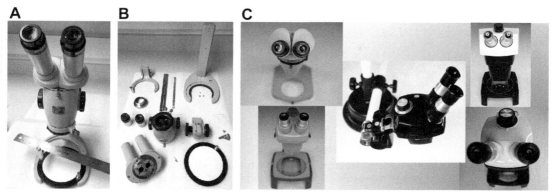

Fig. 2. (*A*) Zeiss STEMI stereo microscope. (*B*) Overlooked Zeiss STEMI stereo microscope disassembled and cleaned by the first author. (*C*) Madison Microneurosurgery Initiative's first 5 stereo microscopes purchased from the University of Wisconsin Surplus With A Purpose (SWAP) online auction.

Once the microscopes were delivered and cleaned, they underwent initial testing by the first author and were then utilized by international research fellows at various levels at the University of Wisconsin–Madison Microneurosurgery Laboratory.

Because these microscopes were bought online, we could not assess their quality and functionality prior to purchase. Thus, we relied on analyzing the condition of the microscopes through photos in the advertisement listings. As we made more purchases, we developed a knack for discerning the quality and functional status from these provided images. Familiarity with certain brands and consistently acquiring microscopes from these known brands also aided us in obtaining properly functioning microscopes. On rare occasions, we had to perform basic repairs after purchase.

Following our initial experience with these microscopes, we expanded our search to include more sources.[12–14] Up to now, we have acquired over 150 stereo microscopes. The acquired stereo microscopes, despite being old, were of high quality and produced by renowned microscopy manufacturers such as Zeiss and Bausch & Lomb. All provided enhanced magnification, high-quality 3 dimensional (3D) views, and a favorable working distance. These very same microscopes, simply by altering their stands, were effectively used in both laboratory settings for live animal surgeries and operating rooms for human surgical procedures.[15–17]

Light Sources

Some of our microscopes were originally equipped with traditional incandescent light sources. To enhance our options, we explored and acquired a variety of illumination solutions from local thrift shops, tech stores, and online platforms. Our collection expanded to include battery powered lights, light-emitting diode (LED) ring light, desk lamps, halogen, (**Fig. 3**A) and xenon light sources (**Fig. 3**B).

Based on our experiences, LED ring lights have emerged as the optimal choice for stereo microscopes. Their advantages include a natural color temperature, minimal heat emission, extended lifespan, reduced power consumption, and a design that is both functional and compact. These lights can be conveniently attached to the underside of the main optical head, offering superior illumination in the viewing area.

In environments where electricity is unavailable, simple battery powered lights prove to be an effective alternative. While halogen and xenon light sources are suitable for more advanced microscopy, their limited availability and higher cost make them impractical for regular use. Additionally, some stereo microscopes feature axial or coaxial illumination; however, we found that this aspect, while beneficial in clinical contexts, is not critical for standard laboratory training, underscoring the versatility and adaptability of our varied illumination solutions.

Instruments

The introduction of operating microscopes used alongside specially designed micro instruments for microsurgery has marked the beginning of a new era in various surgical fields, including neurosurgery. Even before industrial companies crafted specialized microsurgery instruments, various surgical specialties engaged in pioneering microsurgical work using self-designed or adapted instruments.

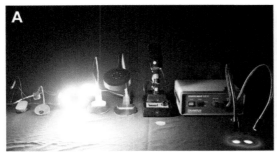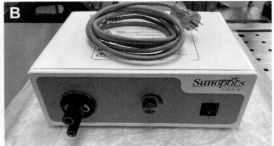

Fig. 3. Various light sources for basic microsurgery laboratory training. (*A*) Battery powered lights, light-emitting diode (LED) ring light, desk lamps, microscope light, and halogen light source. (*B*) Xenon light source. (*B*) (*Used with permission from* Sunoptic Technologies, LLC.)

A critical tool in microvascular training is the fine forceps. Initially, surgeons repurposed jewelry forceps from jewelry stores for this purpose. Julius H. Jacobson II, a pioneer vascular surgeon, developed a simple yet effective test for selecting microsurgical instruments. He showed that any forceps capable of gently extracting a hair follicle from the back of his hand under a microscope, without cutting or slipping, were suitable for microsurgery.[18] To our knowledge, although he did not use the term "tweezers," what he defined as the basic test for jeweler's forceps aligns closely with the function of tweezers, which we use in a similar manner today.

Inspired by Dr. Jacobson's basic test, we procured various tweezer sets online for laboratory training (**Fig. 4**). After evaluating several sets, we identified an excellent and economical choice: a set of 8 forceps, including 6 straight and 2 angled ones, priced at just $9.99, making it an ideal selection for our needs (**Fig. 4**E).

Furthermore, MMI has registered with Hospital Sisters Mission Outreach in Springfield, Illinois, to acquire top-quality, previously owned surgical grade macro/microsurgical instruments.

Training Materials

To facilitate basic microanastomosis training, a variety of materials can be found online. However, in order to simplify the process and ensure global accessibility, we have adopted the BMBTC as our guide for establishing similar microsurgery laboratory training programs in LMICs.

In the BMBTC, the materials utilized include $^1/_4$ inch Penrose drains, silicone tubes of 3 mm and 2 mm, chicken thighs, and sutures of sizes 6-0, 7-0, 9-0, and 10-0. These items are primarily procured from online platforms. For the purpose of training, we use either expired surgical grade or training grade sutures. These materials are generally available in most countries or can be ordered online from abroad.

In certain LMICs, we have not only shared our resources but also sent training materials directly. For other locations, we provided information on our suppliers, enabling them to either order materials online or locate comparable resources within their own countries.

COLLABORATION STRATEGIES AND SELECTION OF DONATION CENTERS

Initially, we utilized our laboratory network to collaborate with health care experts from LMICs, aiding them in acquiring microsurgery laboratory training in their own nations based on individual needs. We provided BTKs to our research fellows from LMICs. As these fellows were trained in our laboratory, they became well-versed in our methods and education style. Upon returning to their countries, they took on the role of remotely instructing other medical professionals from LMICs. Furthermore, they assisted in transporting the training kits back to their countries, significantly reducing one of our major expenses: shipping.

DELIVERY OF KITS

After putting together the kits and selecting partners from LMICs, our focus shifted to identifying the most cost-effective, safe, and reliable way to transfer the kits. Consequently, we identified both individuals and organizations residing or working in those countries to assist us in fulfilling our objectives. So far, our initiatives have impacted 31 facilities in 19 LMICs, involving the distribution of 61 basic microsurgery training kits and 10 sets of advanced microsurgery training kits (**Fig. 5**).

Seventy percent of the kits were distributed by our LMIC research associates. The remaining 30% were delivered through partners such as Solidarity Bridge Neurosurgery and Neurology Institute (SB-NNI) in Paraguay and Bolivia, Duke

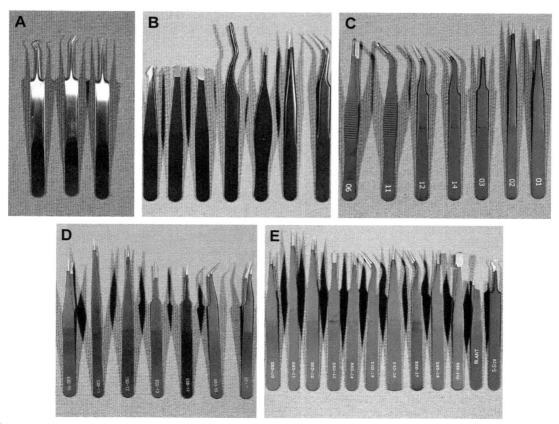

Fig. 4. Various tweezer sets for basic microsurgery laboratory training purchased online for (*A*) $8.99, (*B*) $12.95, (*C*) $9.99, (*D*) $7.99, and (*E*) $$9.99.

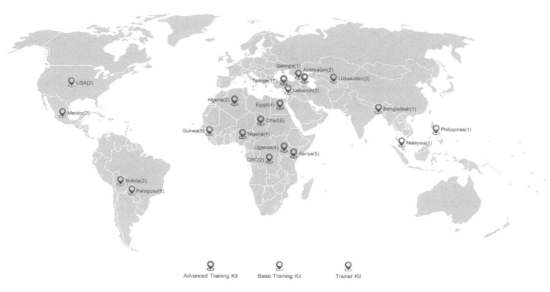

71 Microscopes – 31 Centers – 19 LMICs

Fig. 5. Global distribution of Madison Microneurosurgery Initiative's microsurgery training kit donations to 31 centers in 19 LMICs.

Global Neurosurgery and Neurology in Uganda, and Madison Christ Presbyterian Church in Chad.

In various locations, including Türkiye, Uganda, and Chad, we distributed the kits and training materials through multiple deliveries. Additionally, we handed out some of the kits at the national and international neurosurgery conferences, including the Society for Neuro-Oncology 2022 in Tampa, Florida, Congress of Neurologic Surgeons 2022 in San Francisco, California, American Association of Neurologic Surgeons 2023 in Los Angeles, California, and World Federation of Neurosurgical Societies 2023 in Cape Town, South Africa. These events facilitated direct connections and allowed us to transfer the kits, bypassing the high costs of shipping, even within the United States.

Utilizing these approaches, we managed to minimize our delivery expenses, enabling us to allocate more of our resources toward acquiring additional kits.

TRAINER CENTERS CAPABLE OF LIVE-STREAMED MICROANASTOMOSIS DEMONSTRATION SESSIONS

Our laboratory was outfitted with advanced audiovisual technology equipment used for regular laboratory studies and our annual hands-on courses. This setup comprised a stereoscopic microscope with an integrated camera, a Nikon Z7II professional camera, a Zeiss Pentero surgical microscope equipped with a TrueVision HD 3D camera and station, a computer with an additional external webcam, various tripods, an iPad Pro, 3 liquied-crystal display (LCD) screens, and high-quality lighting equipment (**Fig. 6**).

Apart from our existing setup, we also put together a more compact and user-friendly alternative setup comprised a stereoscopic microscope (**Fig. 7**A) equipped with a beamsplitter, a c-mount camera attachment, and a c-mount camera (**Fig. 7**B). This alternative was not only more compact and easier to use but also significantly more affordable and portable. We sent this same setup to a neurosurgeon, Burak Ozaydin, the former manager of the University of Wisconsin–Madison Microneurosurgery Laboratory, who is now undergoing neurosurgery training at the University of Oklahoma College of Medicine in Oklahoma City. This second center greatly enhanced our capacity for live-streamed demonstrations.

Owing to the compactness and portability of our setup, we utilize it for live demonstrations in-person no-cost hands-on basic microanastomosis courses across 5 countries and at 9 different institutions.

LIVE-STREAMED LECTURES AND MICROANASTOMOSIS DEMONSTRATION SESSIONS

Before dispatching our initial kit to Beirut, Lebanon, we had already planned to conduct live-streamed demonstration sessions with our colleagues, intending to disseminate our know-how and foster the development of microsurgery laboratory training. Following the delivery of the kits, we were all set to start these live-streamed demonstrations. We chose to focus on microanastomosis practice based on the BMBTC, recognizing its essential value and practicality in microsurgical training, as we have noted earlier. We aimed to employ the MOST so that colleagues in LMICs could independently assess their techniques and determine areas for improvement in their following attempts.

From July 18, 2022 to December 7, 2022, we organized 10 live-streamed sessions with colleagues from 4 countries: Türkiye, Paraguay, Lebanon, and Bangladesh (**Table 3**). In Paraguay and Bangladesh, these sessions were coordinated with the support of their neurosurgery societies. Meanwhile, in Türkiye and Lebanon, we arranged these sessions exclusively for 2 trainers in each country.

For each group, we began with lectures on the history of microsurgery, detailing its introduction into neurosurgery, the pioneering works in training laboratories, and its initial clinical applications in the field. We also emphasized the present necessity for this kind of training, which was one of the most critical topics covered. Our experience has shown that trainees who do not fully comprehend the historical background of microsurgery laboratory training, along with its clinical implications and current status, tend to discontinue their training after the initial sessions.

Following the lectures, we held live-streamed sessions which included demonstrations from our bypass training curriculum (**Fig. 8**).

All live-streamed sessions were conducted using Zoom software (Zoom Video Communications, Inc, San Jose, CA). This platform enabled a 2 way real-time participation and dialogue. Crucially, each session was recorded live via Zoom, and these video recordings were shared with participants after each session. The availability of these recordings was vital for reinforcing learning and enabling participants to review the content at their own pace, significantly enhancing the educational value of the series.

TÜRKIYE

We provided a BTK to a neurosurgery resident at Istanbul Faculty of Medicine, Istanbul University.

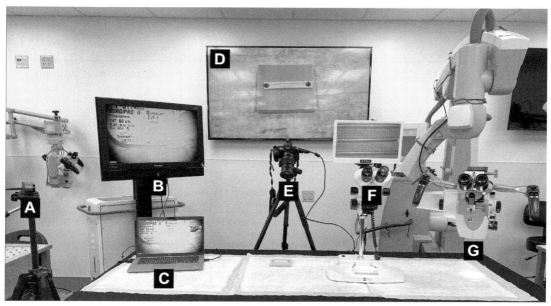

Fig. 6. University of Wisconsin–Madison Microneurosurgery Laboratory audiovisual (AV) setup. Our setup included (*A*) an external webcam, (*B*) a TrueVision HD 3D camera station, (*C*) a computer, (*D*) an LCD screen, (*E*) a Nikon Z7II professional camera, (*F*) a stereoscopic microscope with an integrated camera, and (*G*) a Zeiss Pentero surgical microscope.

At the same time, another resident from Izmir Tepecik Research and Training Hospital reached out to us, expressing his readiness to similar training using his own basic training set and seeking our mentorship. Consequently, we combined the training programs for both residents and arranged 5 live-streamed sessions. Both of the residents completed the initial 3 sections of BMBTC, providing us with their MOST evaluations. This marked the first occasion where we completed and certified such long-distance live-streamed teaching based on the BMBTC and MOST results.

PARAGUAY

In April 2022, we collaborated SB-NNI and president of the Paraguay Neurosurgery Society, in establishing Paraguay's inaugural microneurosurgery laboratory at Hospital Nacional de Itauguá.[19] Our support included sharing our expertise in setting up a microneurosurgery laboratory. As part of this collaboration, we traveled to Des Moines, Iowa, to examine microscopes and to Springfield, Illinois, for selecting and evaluating instruments for the laboratory. Based on our recommendations, SB-NNI managed the procurement

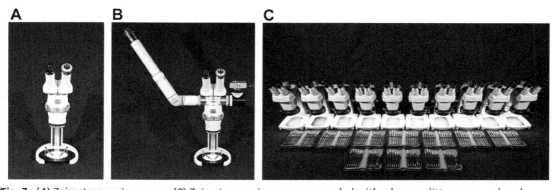

Fig. 7. (*A*) Zeiss stereo microscope. (*B*) Zeiss stereo microscope upgraded with a beamsplitter, monocular observer tube (*left*), and c-mount camera attachment and digital camera (*right*) used for live demonstrations during in-person courses. (*C*) In-person no-cost hands-on microanastomosis course setup of 10 stereo microscopes, 10 LED ring lights, and 10 tweezer sets.

Table 3
Madison microneurosurgery initiative live-streamed teaching sessions

Country	Date	Live-streamed Session
Türkiye	July 18, 2022	Lectures, microsuturing techniques, continuous suturing practice with Penrose drain
	August 25, 2022	End-to-end anastomosis practice with silicone tube
	September 28, 2022	End-to-side and side-to-side anastomosis practice with silicone tube
	November 1, 2022	End-to-end anastomosis practice with chicken vessel
	December 7, 2022	End-to-side and side-to-side anastomosis practice with chicken vessel
Paraguay	July 30, 2022	Lectures
	August 20, 2022	Microsuturing techniques, end-to-end anastomosis practice with silicone tube
Lebanon	August 3, 2022	Lectures, microsuturing techniques, continuous suturing practice with Penrose drain
	December 6, 2022	End-to-end anastomosis practice with silicone tube
Bangladesh	August 27, 2022	Lectures, microsuturing techniques, end-to-end anastomosis practice with silicone tube

and organized the logistics for their secure delivery to Paraguay. Furthermore, we enhanced the laboratory with our donation of 4 Bausch & Lomb Stereo Zoom 4 microscopes, 4 light sources, and a Zeiss operative microscope.

Following the grand opening, we coordinated 2 online live-streamed events in partnership with SB-NNI and the Paraguay Neurosurgery Society. The initial session, a lecture, commenced on July 30, and we followed up with another live-streamed

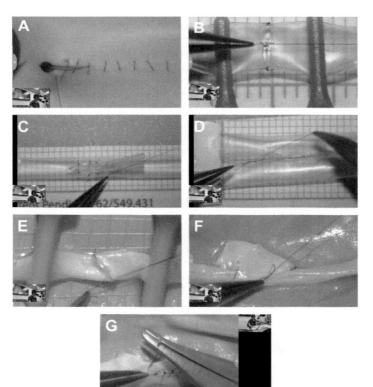

Fig. 8. After the lectures, we held live-streamed sessions that included demonstrations of microsuturing techniques and practices from our bypass training curriculum: (*A*) Continuous suturing practice with 6-0 suture on a Penrose drain, (*B*) end-to-end, (*C*) end-to-side, and (*D*) side-to-side anastomosis demonstrations using 9-0 - sutures on a silicone tube, and (*E*) end-to-end, (*F*) end-to-side, and (*G*) side-to-side anastomosis demonstrations using 10-0 sutures on a chicken vessel.

session on August 20, focusing on microsuturing techniques and end-to-end anastomosis with 3 mm diameter silicone tube using 9-0 suture. A total of 20 participants attended both sessions. In the subsequent days, they arranged a hands-on training session in their microneurosurgery laboratory, where they practiced the techniques that were introduced during the live-streamed session.

LEBANON

MMIs inaugural donation of BTK and training materials was dispatched to the American University of Beirut (AUB), accompanied by one of our research fellows who had successfully completed his BMBTC under our guidance. On August 3, 2022, we organized a live-streamed session with 2 neurosurgery residents from AUB, which included a lecture and hands-on demonstrations in microsuturing techniques, and continuous suturing exercises using on a $^1/_4$ inch Penrose drain with a 6-0 suture. Once both the trainees had completed the initial section of the BMBTC, we hosted another live-streamed event on December 6, 2022, where we demonstrated end-to-end anastomosis using a 3 mm silicone tube with a 9-0 suture. Subsequently, the trainees completed their end-to-end practice with silicone tubes and provided us with their MOST evaluations.

BANGLADESH

Our former research fellow from Bangladesh received a BTK from us as a donation. After his return to Bangladesh, in partnership with the Bangladesh Neurosurgery Society, we conducted a live-streamed lecture on August 27, 2022, attended by 60 participants. After the lecture, we demonstrated microsuturing and end-to-end anastomosis techniques using silicone tubes and 9-0 sutures. Following this, they organized a microanastomosis training session, utilizing our BTK and their existing resources, to practice these techniques.

OTHER LIVE-STREAMED TEACHING OPPORTUNITIES FOR LOW- AND MIDDLE-INCOME COUNTRIES

The Global Visitor Professor Program, initiated by the Foundation for International Education in Neurological Surgery in July 2020, has organized a series of webinars with esteemed experts covering crucial topics such as traumatic brain injury, peripheral nerve surgery, pituitary tumors, spinal cord injuries, and neurotrauma, effectively connecting with neurosurgeons from LMICs through 7 sessions.[20]

Furthermore, in collaboration with the SB-NNI, University of Wisconsin Department of Neurological Surgery started a virtual neurosurgical residency program in December 2022, targeting neurosurgeons in Paraguay and Bolivia. This program has successfully featured 8 comprehensive lectures from the neurosurgeon faculty and alumni, reaching over 60 professionals in these countries.

Last, we disseminated our experiences through online webinar platforms such as Izmir Online and Asian Congress of Neurological Surgeons webinar portals, aiming to raise awareness and motivate others to contribute to neurosurgery in LMICs, similar to our efforts.

IN-PERSON NO-COST HANDS-ON MICROANASTOMOSIS COURSES IN LOW- AND MIDDLE-INCOME COUNTRIES

Beyond our live-streamed remote teaching, as MMI, we introduced a new approach for conducting in-person, hands-on courses in LMICs. Once we gathered a course setup (**Fig. 7**C), we utilized our LMIC connections to organize these hands-on sessions at no cost within their own countries.

To date, we have conducted 9 hands-on microvascular anastomosis courses in 5 countries: Türkiye, Georgia, Azerbaijan, Paraguay, and Mexico, with these sessions being the first of their kind in 7 cities and the inaugural ones in Georgia, Azerbaijan, and Paraguay. Most courses were extensive 1 day events from 9 AM to 6 PM, featuring lectures, live demonstrations, and hands-on practices. In Paraguay, we hosted a 2 day course with additional practices with silicone tubes, while in Mexico, a 3 day course included chicken vessel anastomosis practice (**Table 4**).

At 9 centers, we trained a total of 155 individuals. Unlike similar courses in HICs, our courses in local institutions in LMICs alleviated all the barriers for participants. All courses were offered free of charge. Moreover, we provided participants with our microsurgery training resources and donated several BTKs to these centers, allowing for continued practice postcourse. This was crucial for enabling continued practice and skill development, a benefit not typically available to those attending courses in HICs.

FROM THE MICROSURGICAL LABORATORY TO THE OPERATING ROOM

In our innovative approach, we have provided microsurgery training kits to make microsurgery laboratory techniques accessible in LMICs. Our efforts demonstrated that with sufficient personal

Table 4
Madison Microneurosurgery Initiative in-person no-cost microanastomosis courses

Institution/Number of Participants	Date	Course Outline
Istanbul Medeniyet University, Istanbul, Türkiye/20	January 14, 2023	Lectures Live demonstration and hands-on practice of end-to-end, end-to-side, and side-to-side anastomosis techniques using $\frac{1}{4}$ inch Penrose drain and 6-0 suture
Dicle University, Diyarbakir, Türkiye/16	January 18, 2023	Lectures Live demonstration and hands-on practice of end-to-end, end-to-side, and side-to-side anastomosis techniques using $\frac{1}{4}$ inch Penrose drain and 6-0 suture
Van Yüzüncü Yıl University, Van, Türkiye/12	January 19, 2023	Lectures Live demonstration and hands-on practice of end-to-end, end-to-side, and side-to-side anastomosis techniques using $\frac{1}{4}$ inch Penrose drain and 6-0 suture
Atatürk University, Erzurum, Türkiye/11	January 20, 2023	Lectures Live demonstration and hands-on practice of end-to-end, end-to-side, and side-to-side anastomosis techniques using $\frac{1}{4}$ inch Penrose drain and 6-0 suture
Caucasus Medical Center, Tbilisi, Georgia/14	January 24, 2023	Lectures Live demonstration and hands-on practice of end-to-end, end-to-side, and side-to-side anastomosis techniques using $\frac{1}{4}$ inch Penrose drain and 6-0 suture
Republican Neurosurgery Hospital, Baku, Azerbaijan/15	January 25, 2023	Lectures Live demonstration and hands-on practice of end-to-end, end-to-side, and side-to-side anastomosis techniques using $\frac{1}{4}$ inch Penrose drain and 6-0 suture
Hospital Ingavi IPS, Asuncion, Paraguay/24	June 3–4, 2023	Day 1: Lectures Live demonstration and hands-on practice of end-to-end, end-to-side, and side-to-side anastomosis techniques using $\frac{1}{4}$ inch Penrose drain and 6-0 suture Day 2: Case presentations Live demonstration and hands-on practice of end-to-end, end-to-side, and side-to-side anastomosis techniques with 3 mm and 2 mm silicone tube using 9-0 suture Live demonstration of dissection of chicken thigh and end-to-end anastomosis with chicken vessel using 9-0 suture
Hospital Civil de Guadalajara, Guadalajara, Mexico/21	July 26–29, 2023	Day 1: Lectures Live demonstration and hands-on practice of end-to-end, end-to-side, and side-to-side anastomosis techniques using $\frac{1}{4}$ inch Penrose drain and 6-0 suture Day 2: Case presentations Live demonstration and hands-on practice of end-to-end, end-to-side, and side-to-side anastomosis techniques with 3 and 2 mm silicone tube using 9-0 suture

(continued on next page)

Table 4 (continued)		
Institution/Number of Participants	**Date**	**Course Outline**
		Day 3: Case presentations Live demonstration and hands-on practice of dissection of chicken thigh and end-to-end, end-to-side, and side-to-side anastomosis techniques with chicken vessel using 9-0 suture
Izmir Medical Point Hospital, Izmir, Türkiye/22	August 27, 2023	Lectures End-to-end, end-to-side, and side-to-side anastomosis techniques using $\frac{1}{4}$ inch Penrose drain and 6-0 suture

dedication, this goal could be achieved in 30 centers across 19 LMICs. After establishing these centers, our objective was to teach microtechniques through live-streamed, offline, and in-person support, but we always emphasized that this is just a starting point and not sufficient on its own for applying these techniques in actual surgical operations in the operating room (OR). It is crucial that such assistance efforts be complemented by extensive self-practice to enhance these techniques and maintain the required level of manual dexterity. Only through a combination of comprehensive neuroanatomy knowledge and microsurgical skills can one effectively translate these techniques into the operating room.

In every institution where we conducted live-streamed, offline, and in-person training, we received positive feedback regarding its impact on the trainees' surgical practices in the operating room. In certain centers, following the initiation of laboratory training, our colleagues significantly improved their techniques through extensive laboratory practice and successfully applied these techniques in their surgical procedures. This includes, but is not limited to, performing successful bypass surgeries for moyamoya disease in Tbilisi, Georgia, and Ahmedabad, India, nerve transfers for iatrogenic nerve injuries in Istanbul, Türkiye, and creating arteriovenous fistulas for hemodialysis patients in N'Djamena, Chad.[10] We expect to see an increase in both the quantity and quality of such cases as time progresses.

DISCUSSION

In LMICs, addressing the unmet need for neurosurgical intervention is challenging, with 13.8 of 22.6 million neurologic disorders and injuries requiring surgery, resulting in 5 million unmet cases annually.[21,22] This highlights the need for an additional 23,300 trained neurosurgeons in regions managing 82% of global case volume with only 56% of neurosurgeons.[23] To tackle this, various models and programs have been introduced, including short- and long-term fellowships for neurosurgeons from LMICs, mission trips, Internet-based distance learning (eLearning), and long-term mentorships.[24] These efforts emphasize cost-effective, transferable, and sustainable innovations for training and health care delivery.[25]

Internet-based tools are increasingly recognized for their potential in distance learning, with eLearning offering the advantage of low-cost and on-demand access.[24,26] However, it is recommended to complement eLearning with in-person training to enhance engagement and connection.[27–29] Participants from LMICs face barriers attending congresses in HICs, including geographic, visa, financial, and cultural challenges.[30] A survey by Robertson and colleagues also underscored the unmet need for technical skills workshops and cadaveric laboratories, vital for practical neurosurgical training.[31] This is especially true in locations where other advanced treatment options are limited, making microneurosurgical techniques indispensable for treating neurosurgical pathologies. To become proficient in these microsurgical methods, extensive training in a laboratory setting is essential. Thus, it is highly advised that young professionals spend significant time in training laboratories to acquire knowledge in surgical anatomy and to refine their skills in microsurgical procedures.[32,33] Nevertheless, the availability of training facilities for microsurgery is scarce in both IHCs and LMICs.[31,34,35]

In an innovative effort, we tackled this challenge by supplying neurosurgeons in LMICs with free, cost-effective, and sustainable microsurgery training kits, usable directly at their local institutions and within their own countries. By offering live-streamed instructional sessions, complimentary in-person practical courses, and prerecorded training materials, we have launched self-guided sustainable training programs in 19 LMICs. Up to this point, the MMI has been significantly supported by the personal contributions of the first author, exceeding $25,000, and further augmented by a generous $1000 donation from one of the senior authors (MKB). These funds have covered essential expenses such as microscopes, lighting equipment, instruments, shipping, complimentary in-person practical courses, and other associated costs.

SUMMARY

Modern technology has transformed neurosurgical education, paving the way for neurosurgical care in LMICs and enabling a standard of neurosurgical service that was previously unattainable in these areas. Our innovative method suggests that the combination of donating microsurgery training kits and providing live-streamed instruction for microvascular surgery training makes remote microsurgical education feasible. We believe that this new strategy will be instrumental in bridging the gap in teaching and spreading microsurgical techniques, especially in LMICs where there is a critical need for such skills.

CLINICS CARE POINTS

- Microsurgery laboratory training is crucial worldwide, especially in LMICs due to the scarcity of advanced surgical facilities. Establishing localized training laboratories can significantly enhance the surgical skills necessary to improve patient outcomes in these regions.

- The MMI has pioneered the provision of essential microsurgery skills by donating specialized training sets to LMICs, directly addressing the gap in surgical education and infrastructure.

- MMI's novel approach combines set donations with comprehensive support mechanisms, including live-streamed, offline, and in-person sessions. This model ensures a robust training environment that adapts to various educational and resource settings in LMICs.

- Alongside traditional methods, the use of alternative remote teaching tools such as offline video demonstration sources, interactive webinars, and live-streamed demonstration sessions can enhance learning flexibility and

accessibility, catering to diverse learner needs and contexts.

- Implementing such a multifaceted and adaptable teaching strategy for microsurgery in LMICs is pivotal, offering a sustainable solution to bridge educational gaps and foster local expertise in essential surgical skills.

DISCLOSURE

The authors have nothing to disclose.

FUNDING

Up to this point, the MMI has been significantly supported by the personal contributions of the first author, exceeding $25,000, and further augmented by a generous $1000 donation from one of the senior authors (MKB).

REFERENCES

1. Yaşargil MG. Microsurgery: applied to neurosurgery. Thieme; 1969.

2. Donaghy RP, Yaşargil MG. Micro-vascular surgery: report of first conference, October 6-7, 1966, mary Fletcher Hospital. Burlington, Vermont: CV Mosby Company; 1967.

3. Irwin A, Valentine N, Brown C, et al. The commission on social determinants of health: Tackling the social roots of health inequities. Editorial Material. PLoS Med 2006;3(6):749–51. e106.

4. Sayyahmelli S, Kessely YC, Chen X, et al. From Ibni Sina (Avicenna) to Present, History of International Fellowship and Observership: University of Wisconsin-Madison Experience. Turk Neurosurg 2020;30(2):159–62.

5. Jacobson JH, Wallman LJ, Schumacher GA, et al. Microsurgery as an aid to middle cerebral artery endarterectomy. Microsurgery 1992;13(3):112–8.

6. Jacobson JH. The early days of microsurgery in Vermont. Mt Sinai J Med 1997;64(3):160–3.

7. Yaşargil MG. A legacy of microneurosurgery: Memoirs, lessons, and axioms. Neurosurgery 1999; 45(5):1025–92.

8. Donaghy RM. The history of microsurgery in neurosurgery. Clin Neurosurg 1979;26:619–25.

9. Yaşargil MG. The advent of microsurgery. Mt Sinai J Med 1997;64(3):164–5.

10. Keles A, Cancela AA, Moussalem CK, et al. A Novel Approach for Free, Affordable, and Sustainable Microsurgery Laboratory Training for Low- and Middle-Income Countries: University of Wisconsin-Madison Microneurosurgery Laboratory Experience. Neurosurgery 2024;1–13.

11. University of Wisconsin-Madison SWAP Online Auction. UW SWAP. Available at: https://swapauction.wisc.edu/. [Accessed 29 June 2023].

12. U.S. General Services Administration. GSA Auctions. Available at: https://gsaauctions.gov/auctions/home. [Accessed 29 June 2023].

13. Wisconsin Surplus. Wisconsin Surplus Online Auction. Available at: https://wisconsinsurplus.com/. [Accessed 29 June 2023].

14. Auctions HiBid. HiBid Wisconsin. Accessed June 29, 2023. hibid.com/" title="https://wisconsin. hibid.com/">https://wisconsin. hibid.com/.

15. Silveira L, Duffy L, Adams D, et al. Great Hospitals: The History of Neurosurgery at the University of Vermont Medical Center–A Macroscopic Examination of Microscope-Savvy Pioneers. World Neurosurg 2023; 174:146–56.

16. Terzis JK. History of Microsurgery. Lulu 2011;34-39: 240–71.

17. Company AO. The New AO Surgical Microscope. Trans Am Acad Ophthalmol Otolaryngol 1959;63.

18. Drotar DL. Micro-surgery: revolution in the operating room. Beaufort Books; 1981.

19. Bridge S. Training the Next Generation of Neuro Specialists. 2023. Available at: https://www.solidarity bridge.org/blog/training-the-next-generation-of-neuro-specialists. [Accessed 13 November 2023].

20. FIENS. Virtual Visiting Professor. 2024. Available at: https://fiens.org/education/virtual-visiting-professor/. [Accessed 15 January 2024].

21. Meara JG, Leather AJM, Hagander L, et al. Global Surgery 2030: Evidence and solutions for achieving health, welfare, and economic development. Article. Surgery 2015;158(1):3–6.

22. Fuller AT, Barkley A, Du R, et al. Global neurosurgery: a scoping review detailing the current state of international neurosurgical outreach. Review. J Neurosurg 2021;134(4):1316–24.

23. Dewan MC, Rattani A, Fieggen G, et al. Global neurosurgery: the current capacity and deficit in the provision of essential neurosurgical care. Executive Summary of the Global Neurosurgery Initiative at the Program in Global Surgery and Social Change. Article. J Neurosurg 2019;130(4): 1055–64.

24. Almeida JP, Velasquez C, Karekezi C, et al. Global neurosurgery: models for international surgical education and collaboration at one university. Article. Neurosurg Focus 2018;45(4):E5.

25. Warf BC. "Who Is My Neighbor?" Global Neurosurgery in a Non-Zero-Sum World. Editorial Material. World Neurosurg 2015;84(6):1547–9.

26. Blankstein U, Dakurah T, Bagan M, et al. Structured online neurosurgical education as a novel method of education delivery in the developing world. ; Research Support, Non-U.S. Gov't. World Neurosurg 2011;76(3–4):224–30.

27. Liang KE, Bernstein I, Kato Y, et al. Enhancing Neurosurgical Education in Low- and Middle-income Countries: Current Methods and New Advances. Review. Neurol Med -Chir 2016;56(11):709–15.

28. Sedney CL, Siu J, Rosseau G, et al. International Neurosurgical Volunteerism: A Temporal, Geographic, and Thematic Analysis of Foundation for International Education in Neurological Surgery Volunteer Reports. World Neurosurg 2014;82(6).

29. Shrime MG, Bickler SW, Alkire BC, et al. Global burden of surgical disease: an estimation from the provider perspective. Letter. Lancet Global Health 2015;3:S8–9.

30. Sharma V, Boyke A, Shlobin NA, et al. Characteristics of global neurosurgery sessions: a retrospective analysis of major international neurosurgical conferences. World Neurosurg 2021;150:E790–3.

31. Robertson FC, Gnanakumar S, Karekezi C, et al. The World Federation of Neurosurgical Societies Young Neurosurgeons Survey (Part II): Barriers to Professional Development and Service Delivery in Neurosurgery. World neurosurgery: X 2020;8:100084.

32. Yaşargil MG. From the microsurgical laboratory to the operating theatre. Editorial Material. Acta Neurochir 2005;147(5):465–8.

33. Yaşargil M. Microneurosurgery: Principles, applications, and training. In: Sindou M, editor. Practical handbook of neurosurgery: from leading neurosurgeons. Springer Verlag; 2009. p. 3–30.

34. Sarpong K, Fadalla T, Garba DL, et al. Access to training in neurosurgery (Part 1): Global perspectives and contributing factors of barriers to access. Brain & spine 2022;2:100900.

35. Gnanakumar S, Abou El Ela Bourquin B, Robertson FC, et al. The World Federation of Neurosurgical Societies Young Neurosurgeons Survey (Part I): Demographics, Resources, and Education. World neurosurgery: X 2020;8:100083.

Partnering with Foundations, Philanthropy, and Universities with Programs Supported by Local Physicians and Eventually Local Physicians Taking Ownership

Radzi Hamzah, MD, MPH[a],*, Kate Bunch, MD[b],
Moody Qureshi, MBChB MMed (Surgery), FCS-ECSA, FRCSEd(SN)[c],
Kee B. Park, MD, MPH[a], Michael M. Haglund, MD, PhD, Med, MACM[d],
Robert J. Dempsey, MD[b]

KEYWORDS

- Global neurosurgery • Partnership • Capacity • High-income country
- Low-income and middle-income country

KEY POINTS

- Transformative partnerships between various stakeholders, including foundations, philanthropic organizations, and universities, are crucial for evolving short-term medical missions into sustainable, locally led neurosurgical programs in low-income and middle-income countries (LMICs).
- Long-term educational exchanges and training programs, supported by innovative digital platforms, are essential in building local capacities and enhancing global neurosurgical competency, thereby promoting self-sufficiency in neurosurgical care.
- Research collaborations and the development of sustainable technology solutions are key to advancing neurosurgical care, with a focus on aligning with the specific needs and contexts of LMICs to ensure relevance and effectiveness.
- Empowering local physicians to take leadership roles in neurosurgical programs and ensuring culturally competent care are fundamental in building patient trust and effectively delivering neurosurgical services in diverse cultural settings.

[a] Program in Global Surgery and Social Change, Department of Global Health and Social Medicine, Harvard Medical School, Boston, MA 02115, USA; [b] Department of Neurological Surgery, University of Wisconsin-Madison, 600 Highland Avenue, K4/8 CSC, Box 8660, Madison, WI 53792, USA; [c] Department of Neurosurgery, 1st Floor, Aga Khan Hospital, P.O. Box 76553 3rd Parklands Avenue, Nairobi, Kenya; [d] Department of Neurological Surgery, Duke University, 40 Duke Medicine Cir, Durham, NC 27710, USA
* Corresponding author.
E-mail address: radzihamzahMD@gmail.com

Neurosurg Clin N Am 35 (2024) 465–474
https://doi.org/10.1016/j.nec.2024.05.008
1042-3680/24/© 2024 Elsevier Inc. All rights are reserved, including those for text and data mining, AI training, and similar technologies.

INTRODUCTION

The World Federation of Neurosurgical Societies (WFNS) Global Neurosurgery Committee defines global neurosurgery as the clinical and public health practice of neurosurgery with the primary purpose of ensuring timely, safe, and affordable neurosurgical care to all who need it.[1] This field emphasizes neurosurgery's vital significance in the larger context of global health and argues for its complete inclusion into global health development goals.[1,2]

Tracing the growth of global neurosurgery illustrates a transforming journey from its early days of short-term trips to a current landscape characterized by systematic, strategic approaches. This paradigm shift was significantly affected by landmark events and publications, including the pivotal Bogota Declaration in 2016 and the seminal paper by the Lancet Commission on Global Surgery in 2015.[2–6] These milestones highlighted the global surgery community's collective agreement on the importance of addressing significant inequities in surgical including neurosurgical care, particularly in low-income and middle-income countries (LMICs).

Despite significant advances, the current scenario in worldwide neurosurgical outreach faces tremendous hurdles. An estimated 5 billion individuals do not have access to necessary surgical care, with a significant gap of around 5 million neurosurgery procedures per year.[2,6,7] This unmet need highlights the significant scarcity of neurosurgeons, which is expected to be filled by an extra 20,000 practitioners.[7,8]

In response to these obstacles, innovative partnership models have arisen, best exemplified by the concept of "twinning" between institutions from different economic climates.[9,10] Such collaborations involve a wide range of activities, including surgical camps, educational programs, research partnerships, and the construction of residency and fellowship programs, all with the goal of strengthening local capacities and supporting long-term improvement in neurosurgical care.[4,9–13]

These programs are fueled by foundational support, philanthropic contributions, and academic relationships.[4,9,13,14] This multimodal support provides local physicians with the necessary knowledge and abilities, allowing them to lead and sustain these programs. This empowerment is consistent with the overarching goals of global health, which promote autonomy, adaptation, and resilience in health care systems worldwide.

As this article progresses, it will discuss the crucial importance of partnership in the continued evolution of global neurosurgery. Through the perspective of collaboration and solidarity, the discipline is gradually evolving toward a future in which neurosurgical treatment transcends geographic and socioeconomic barriers, representing the principle of fairness in health for everyone.

THE POWER OF PARTNERSHIP

Within the field of global neurosurgery, the natural collaborative nature of partnerships serves as a source of optimism, greatly enhancing resources, expanding influence, and promoting lasting improvements in neurosurgical care. Partnerships bring together a variety of abilities, experience, and resources to generate a powerful force in addressing the deep-rooted difficulties of global neurosurgery. Throughout history, these cooperative endeavors have witnessed a diverse range of interactions with universities, with each collaboration characterized by its distinct structure and execution.

The Evolution from Short-Term Trips

Initially, the mission to bridge gaps in neurosurgical care often took the form of short-term humanitarian missions by surgeons from high-income countries (HICs). These visits, typically characterized by brief, intensive surgical camps LMICs, were seen as a cost-effective way to deliver immediate care.[15] However, despite their immediate benefits, these short-term engagements fell short of laying the groundwork for sustainable neurosurgical programs.[16] They offered little in the way of building local capacities that could adapt to the unique cultural, economic, and medical landscapes of LMICs.[16]

Beyond Short-Term Solutions: Fostering Sustainable Growth

An optimal next step after these brief commitments is to establish a lasting framework in which local surgeons are not only provided the necessary resources and training, but also empowered to share this knowledge with others, creating a self-sufficient network of neurosurgical expertise. Nevertheless, this shift is filled with difficulties, such as inadequate infrastructure, a lack of technical assistance, the regular upkeep of equipment, the absence of defined treatment guidelines, and reduced physician trust due to an excessive number of cases.[9,12,17]

The donation of medical equipment and technology, while invaluable, introduces complexities, particularly when the capacity for maintenance and repair is lacking.[18] Coupled with the fact that much of the donated equipment is not tailored to the specific needs and conditions of LMICs, this has led to a significant portion of medical devices being nonoperational, as evidenced by reports indicating that up to 40% of such equipment in Africa is out of service.[12,19] The engagement of HIC collaborators in on-the-ground missions offers a more nuanced perspective of the resource landscape in LMICs, enabling a more informed approach to technology donations that are both relevant and sustainable.[5,11]

Participating directly in LMIC settings enables HIC neurosurgeons to get firsthand understanding of the distinct clinical difficulties and requirements for patient treatment in these areas. This immersive experience not only enhances comprehension of the local medical environment but also ensures that contributions are accurately tailored to the actual requirements of the people in LMICs, hence increasing the effectiveness and influence of global neurosurgical partnerships.

DIFFERENT AREAS OF PARTNERSHIP
Enhancing Global Neurosurgical Competency via Collaborative Education and Hosting in Neurosurgical Training

The global expansion of neurosurgical care heavily depends on collaboration partnerships with academic institutions, characterized by diverse and inventive concepts and implementations.[20,21] These collaborations are essential for enabling neurosurgeons and trainees to go to HICs for advanced training, allowing them to learn and experience new surgical methods and expand their knowledge of neurosurgical practices.[10,13,20,22] These exchanges promote enduring mentorships and collaborative networks that last long after the trainees have returned to their home countries.

Key programs and opportunities
The CNS Foundation's International Observership Program distinguishes itself via its dedication to education, providing scholarships to cover the educational and living costs of highly skilled residents.[9] This program offers a 3 to 6 month opportunity to fully engage in renowned neurosurgery programs, enabling participants to directly experience and learn about the most recent surgical developments.[9] Additional esteemed establishments, such Harvard, Icahn School of Medicine at Mount Sinai, Duke, and UPMC, provide comparable prospects, each with its distinct emphasis and length. These programs are crucial for earners, granting them access to high-quality training environments either for free or at a small cost, greatly improving their skills.

Another example is through the Foundation for International Education in Neurosurgery (FIENS). FIENS contributes significantly by providing Bassett and Clack Family fellowships, which aid in the education of residents and neurosurgeons from other nations.[9,23] FIENS facilitates up to 10 global neurosurgery fellowships each year to promote educational collaboration and resource sharing among countries with varying income levels.[9,23] This aligns with FIENS' concept of encouraging systemic change via education.[23] This method not only enhances the impact of FIENS but also contributes to communal endeavors in attaining local health goals.

Limitations and challenges of hosting programs
Despite the evident benefits of these programs for individual growth, they have difficulties in contributing to the greater purpose of developing sustainable neurosurgical practices in LMICs. Returnees frequently have difficulties in using their recently acquired knowledge because of the significant discrepancy in resources and equipment between their home countries and HICs.[24] This discrepancy prompts inquiries on the pragmatic implementation of the abilities obtained elsewhere within their specific health care settings.

Furthermore, there is apprehension that these programs can unintentionally provide learners with abilities that rely on resources and technology that are not readily available in their own homes, so restricting the practicality of their training. The possibility of "brain drain," in which clinicians choose to stay in HICs after their training, adds another layer of complexity to the situation; however, there is a lack of solid data connecting neurosurgical fellowships or observership to this trend.[5,25]

Embracing south–south collaboration for neurosurgical advancement
The development of WFNS Training Centers in Sub-Saharan Africa has significantly augmented the quantity of neurosurgeons in the region, resulting in a substantial number of them returning to their home countries to actively participate in local training initiatives.[26–28] The WFNS Rabat Training Center, founded through a collaboration with Mohamed V University and the Faculty of Medicine and Pharmacy of Rabat, has taught 58 trainees from roughly 18 Sub-Saharan countries since its start in 2002.[26,27,29] The center demonstrates the effectiveness of cooperative training initiatives, with support from many partners.

WFNS's certification of additional centers in Algeria, Kenya, and Senegal underscores the expanding network of neurosurgical training programs in Sub-Saharan Africa.[27–29] The establishment of a WFNS regional alumni association seeks to enhance the cohesion of these endeavors, enabling a seamless interchange of information within the African neurosurgical community.

Engaging in partnerships with nearby surgical teams, universities, and regional surgical societies is crucial for maintaining Continuing Medical Education and fostering professional growth. The Continental Association of African Neurosurgical Societies provides a platform for education led by Africans, creating a supportive environment for neurosurgeons in the continent through local and regional educational activities.[28,30] Supported by esteemed institutions like the West African College of Surgeons and the College of Surgeons of East, Central, and Southern Africa, this model highlights the significance of local training in promoting the progress of neurosurgical treatment throughout the continent.

Research Collaborations: Enhancing Global Neurosurgical Care via Mutual Benefits and Collaborative Models

Partnerships between universities in LMICs and HICs in the field of research offer substantial benefits for both parties involved.[21] An example of such advantageous collaborations is the Global Neuro-Surg Research Collaborative, which connects the Neurological Surgery Department of Oregon Health and Science Institute with institutes in nations such as India and Uganda.[31,32] This collaboration is dedicated to researching traumatic brain injuries in various economic contexts, emphasizing the worldwide scope of neurosurgical difficulties. Other collaborations, for example, the Duke in Uganda program have led to over 100 publications in the last decade many with Uganda colleagues as the key contributors and authors.[12]

The significance of conducting research that is both contextual and evidence-based cannot be overstated. The core of these collaborations resides in their capacity to generate research that is grounded in empirical evidence and tailored to the specific neurosurgical conditions seen in LMICs. LMICs, in contrast to HICs, frequently encounter unique diseases and limitations in resources, which require customized approaches for research and health care. Nevertheless, it is imperative to guarantee that these research endeavors are in accordance with the interests of partners in LMICs and fairly recognize their contributions. A survey conducted among trainees at the Makerere College of Health Sciences in Uganda unveiled a deficiency in synchronizing research with local goals and acknowledging the efforts of local researchers, emphasizing the necessity for more comprehensive research models.[33]

Hence, addressing these discrepancies in neurosurgical publications is imperative for comprehensive research. The worldwide dissemination of neurosurgical studies additionally demonstrates the discrepancy in research contributions, with a notable lack of representation from authors in LMICs.[34,35] This disparity not only demonstrates the disparity in resources, but also underscores the significance of cultivating research settings that promote and facilitate the involvement of neurosurgeons from LMICs.[34,35] The BOOTStraP initiative in Colombia is a project that seeks to provide guidelines for managing traumatic brain injuries, specifically tailored to the available resources.[34,35] This project is supported by international institutions and serves as an outstanding example of how collaborative efforts can address these gaps.[34,35]

Toward Sustainable and Equitable Partnerships

For these collaborations to be really efficient and enduring, they must not only entail the exchange of resources and skills, but also guarantee that the research undertaken is directly applicable to the requirements of LMIC settings.[34,35] HIC partners, with their sophisticated data gathering methods, randomized controlled trials, and expertise in developing guidelines, need to cooperate closely with LMIC surgeons who are experienced in operating under constrained resource conditions.[34,35] By prioritizing inquiries relevant to regional customs and formulating pragmatic recommendations for specific contexts, such partnerships can have a substantial influence on the worldwide neurosurgical community.

Leveraging Online Education and Collaborative Partnerships in Neurosurgery

The incorporation of digital platforms in neurosurgery education is a notable advancement in tackling worldwide educational inequalities.[25,36] The partnership between the University of Toronto and the Association of Surgeons of East Africa, as demonstrated by the Ptolemy project, highlights the capacity of digital resources to offer extensive availability of medical literature to health care professionals in underdeveloped areas.[37] This endeavor showcases the efficacy of digital platforms in augmenting knowledge while keeping operational expenses to a minimum, therefore establishing a precedent for similar educational programs globally.[37]

The feedback from participants in the Ptolemy project highlights the significant and positive effect of digital access for health care practice and educational advancement, despite the relatively expensive Internet connectivity in certain areas.[37] Nevertheless, the task persists to duplicate the tangible and all-encompassing encounter of practical surgical instruction using digital methods.[9]

Innovative Hybrid Models and Global Alliances

Hybrid educational methods have been implemented to reconcile the disparity between digital and physical learning experiences, by combining online learning with in-person instruction.[9,38] The NeuroKids program employs a combination of initial in-person instruction and subsequent virtual coaching to facilitate ongoing skill development and establish a self-sustaining educational cycle.[9] Similarly, the Seattle Science Foundation's use of top-notch video modules alongside fellowship possibilities showcases how hybrid models may offer a holistic learning experience.[39]

The effectiveness of international partnerships, like the NED Foundation's projects in Tanzania/Zanzibar and the Meditech Foundation's efforts in Colombia, further demonstrates the influence of tailored educational programs in improving neurosurgical treatment within local health care systems.[12,39,40] These initiatives enhance both clinical abilities and play a vital role in establishing neurosurgical guidelines and research capacities in LMICs.

Overcoming Obstacles in Digital Education

The shift toward digital and hybrid learning models poses various hurdles, such as technological difficulties and the intricacies of coordinating virtual events.[41] For the successful execution of virtual neurosurgical education, it is vital to guarantee uninterrupted access to digital platforms, offer alternate methods for delivering content, and establish good communication with speakers.[38,41]

InterSurgeon is a virtual platform that facilitates collaborative partnerships within the global surgery community, providing access to essential information and technical tools.[39,42,43] It functions as a valuable platform for facilitating connections between partners for worldwide neurosurgical fellowships and improving the accessibility of standardized resources and augmented reality applications.[39,42,43]

The Toronto SickKids fellowship program is another outstanding example, as it welcomes international fellows and is financially supported by hospital divisions.[39] Notwithstanding obstacles related to licensure, visa matters, and cultural disparities, this initiative has effectively established a global network of proficient neurosurgeons who make valuable contributions to neurosurgical health care in their respective nations.[9]

Future Directions in Virtual Training

The introduction of a clinical global neurosurgical hybrid fellowship, which includes significant virtual elements, presents an innovative method for broadening educational outreach. Virtual platforms are unable to completely duplicate the complexities of surgical training, but they are extremely beneficial for instructing on theoretic issues such as operative anatomy, patient selection, and pre-operative and post-operative care.[9] Utilizing remote mentorship and flipped classroom techniques can optimize the learning experience, equipping trainees with the necessary skills for the practical parts of neurosurgery.[9,44]

Examples like the initiatives by the Society of Haitian Neuroscientists and the global neurosurgery fellowship by Universidad del Valle in Colombia illustrate diverse approaches to neurosurgical education across different regions.[9] These initiatives aim to develop educational models that are resilient, inclusive, and effective, addressing current disparities and fostering a more interconnected and skilled global neurosurgical workforce.

ENGAGING DIVERSE STAKEHOLDERS IN NEUROSURGERY PARTNERSHIPS
Foundations: Catalysts for Neurosurgical Progress

Foundations are vital in driving forward neurosurgical initiatives by providing essential funding for research, education, and clinical programs. Their contributions are crucial across the spectrum of neurosurgical care in both HICs and LMICs. For example, the Barrow Neurological Foundation supports a wide range of neurosurgical specializations, from traumatic brain injury to neuromuscular diseases, enhancing the scope of care available.[45] Similarly, the Neurosurgery Research and Education Foundation offers substantial fellowship grants, fostering the development of future neurosurgical leaders.[46,47]

Internationally, programs like as the Global Neurosurgery Initiative, led by the Program in Global Surgery and Social Change at Harvard Medical School, strive to tackle the global burden of neurosurgical issues through research and activism.[48] The CNS Foundation demonstrates this worldwide endeavor by providing financing for diverse neurosurgical developments, showcasing the comprehensive support system for the progress of neurosurgery.[9,49]

Collaborations with foundations like the Duke Global Neurosurgery and Neurology and the FIENS underscore the importance of aligning with organizations that share a commitment to advancing neurosurgical care.[9,10] Successful partnerships can lead to significant advancements in neurosurgical clinics through financial support, resource allocation, and shared expertise.

Regional initiatives, such as the ones backed by the Palestine Children's Relief Fund in the Middle East and the joint endeavors in Ethiopia involving the University of Bergen and FIENS, illustrate how focused assistance can strengthen local neurosurgical capabilities and boost patient results.[9]

Philanthropy: a Strategic Force in Global Neurosurgery

Engaging philanthropic entities requires a strategic approach that highlights the transformative impact of philanthropic support on neurosurgical care. Crafting a compelling narrative that demonstrates the critical need for enhanced neurosurgical services is key to attracting philanthropic involvement. This narrative should articulate how philanthropic contributions can support research endeavors, staff recruitment, and the acquisition of crucial equipment.

The CNS Foundation exemplifies philanthropy in practice by fostering international cooperation among neurosurgeons and providing assistance to pioneering initiatives that tackle worldwide neurosurgical needs.[39,50] The partnership with organizations such as the World Federation of Neurosurgical Societies and the National Institute for Health Research Global Health Research Group on Neurotrauma demonstrates the joint endeavor to progress the area of neurosurgery.[39]

Innovative fundraising models, such as venture philanthropy, offer new avenues for engaging philanthropists by fostering partnerships between health organizations, academia, and industry.[51,52] These collaborations can accelerate the development of new treatments and technologies, furthering the impact of philanthropy in neurosurgery.[52]

Prominent philanthropic organizations, such as the Bill & Melinda Gates Foundation, demonstrate the significant role philanthropy can play in addressing global health challenges.[53,54] Their substantial investments in health care initiatives underscore the potential for philanthropic funding to make a meaningful difference in global neurosurgical care.

Private–Public Partnerships: Exploring New Frontiers in Funding

Private–public partnerships (PPPs) are a valuable but not fully utilized option in the field of global neurosurgery. They provide a framework for combining the resources and innovative capabilities of the private sector with the accessibility and regulatory control of the public sector.[14] Although PPPs have played a crucial role in numerous global health projects, their promise in the field of neurosurgery has not been fully utilized.[14] These collaborations have the potential to expedite the establishment of neurosurgical infrastructure, developments in technology, and training initiatives, especially LMICs where the demand is most urgent.

The adoption of PPP models from other health sectors could revolutionize the way neurosurgical services are delivered and expanded, especially in regions with limited resources.[55] By exploring PPPs as a viable funding mechanism, the neurosurgical community can unlock new possibilities for collaboration, innovation, and sustainable development in neurosurgical care and education globally.

BENEFITS OF INDEPENDENCE CULTURAL COMPETENCY

The need for local, independent neurosurgical care is clear. Improving access to care in LMICs via local, independent care is not only moral and ethical, and economical, but having neurosurgeons of the same background, ethnicity, and culture as their patients lends itself to culturally sensitive care and patient–physician trust.[56] In the United States, there has been a wealth of literature suggesting that patients with physicians who share their same race, ethnicity, culture, or background are more likely to be more receptive to their recommendations,[57] view them more favorably,[57] be more likely to adhere to recommended medication regimens,[58] are associated with improved infant mortality,[59] or even understanding medical information presented to them.[60] Should these associations follow cultures outside of the United States, it becomes all the more important to have strong cultural representation in treating physicians from the groups of people in a particular patient population. In some cultures, in Africa, for example, neurologic disease has been attributed to sorcery or other metaphysical characteristics causing stigmatization and potential impacts in seeking care.[61,62] Visiting physicians from other cultures may have a hard time relating to such beliefs or navigating questions that explore the interplay between those cultural beliefs, for which they may have little understanding, and the medical information they are attempting to impart. It is possible that regardless of their communication skills, fund of knowledge, or bedside manner, they might be unable to fully connect with some patients and be able to counsel them effectively. While there is no, to our knowledge, literature linking the cultural and racial concordance of patients and providers in LMICs to superior outcomes, the ability of local physicians and surgeons to provide care in the context of the community of which they are a part of may be critical to patients fully understanding their own needs.

SUMMARY

In conclusion, the article underscores the necessity of a collaborative, multi-faceted approach in global neurosurgery to overcome the challenges of access and quality of care in underserved regions. By fostering strategic partnerships, prioritizing education and training, and leveraging innovative technologies, the global neurosurgery community can make significant strides toward equitable neurosurgical care worldwide. These efforts not only aim to fill the current gaps in care and expertise but also to empower local health systems with the resilience and capacity to address future neurosurgical needs independently, ensuring that neurosurgical care is accessible and equitable for all who need it, regardless of geographic or economic barriers.

CLINICS CARE POINTS

- Transformative Partnerships: The importance of partnerships between foundations, philanthropic organizations, and universities in evolving short-term medical missions into sustainable, locally-led neurosurgical programs in low- and middle-income countries (LMICs).

- Educational Exchanges and Training Programs: Long-term educational exchanges and training programs, supported by innovative digital platforms, are essential in building local capacities and enhancing global neurosurgical competency, thereby promoting self-sufficiency in neurosurgical care.

- Research Collaborations: Collaborative research and the development of sustainable technology solutions are key to advancing neurosurgical care, focusing on the specific needs and contexts of LMICs to ensure relevance and effectiveness.

- Empowerment of Local Physicians: Empowering local physicians to take leadership roles in neurosurgical programs and ensuring culturally competent care are fundamental in building patient trust and effectively delivering neurosurgical services in diverse cultural settings.

- Sustainable Growth Beyond Short-Term Solutions: Establishing lasting frameworks where local surgeons are provided with necessary resources and training, enabling them to create a self-sufficient network of neurosurgical expertise.

- Local Competency and Cultural Sensitivity: Local, independent neurosurgical care is crucial for providing culturally sensitive care and building patient-physician trust, particularly in LMICs.

- Collaborative Educational Models: Partnerships with academic institutions facilitate neurosurgeons and trainees from LMICs to gain advanced training in high-income countries (HICs), promoting enduring mentorships and collaborative networks.

- Challenges of Hosting Programs: Addressing the discrepancies in resources and equipment between HICs and LMICs, and mitigating the risk of "brain drain" where clinicians might stay in HICs after training.

- South-South Collaboration: The development of training centers in Sub-Saharan Africa has significantly increased the number of neurosurgeons in the region, with many returning to their home countries to participate in local training initiatives.

- Digital Education and Hybrid Models: The use of digital platforms and hybrid educational models to tackle educational inequalities, providing extensive access to medical literature and continuous skill development.

- Engagement with Diverse Stakeholders: The role of foundations, philanthropic organizations, and private-public partnerships in driving forward neurosurgical initiatives by providing essential funding, research support, and clinical programs.

- Overcoming Obstacles in Digital Education: Ensuring uninterrupted access to digital platforms, alternative content delivery methods, and effective communication for successful virtual neurosurgical education.

- Future Directions: Embracing innovative approaches like hybrid fellowships with significant virtual elements to broaden educational outreach and optimize learning experiences for neurosurgical trainees.

DISCLOSURE

No financial disclosure.

REFERENCES

1. Kanmounye US, Esene IN. Letter: Global Neurosurgery Scope and Practice. Neurosurgery Practice 2021;2(3):okab025.

2. Park KB, Johnson WD, Dempsey RJ. Global Neurosurgery: The Unmet Need. World Neurosurg 2016; 88:32–5.

3. Gomez MG, Arynchyna-Smith A, Ghotme KA, et al. Global Neurosurgery at the 76th World Health Assembly (2023): First Neurosurgery-driven Resolution Calls for Micronutrient Fortification to Prevent Spina Bifida. World Neurosurg 2024. https://doi.org/10.1016/j.wneu.2024.01.089.

4. Uche EO, Sundblom J, Uko UK, et al. Global neurosurgery over a 60-year period: Conceptual foundations, time reference, emerging Co-ordinates and prospects for collaborative interventions in low and middle income countries. Brain Spine 2022;2:101187.

5. Haglund MM, Fuller AT. Global neurosurgery: innovators, strategies, and the way forward: JNSPG 75th Anniversary Invited Review Article. J Neurosurg 2019;131(4):993–9.

6. Meara JG, Leather AJM, Hagander L, et al. Global Surgery 2030: evidence and solutions for achieving health, welfare, and economic development. Lancet 2015;386(9993):569–624.

7. Dewan MC, Rattani A, Fieggen G, et al. Global neurosurgery: the current capacity and deficit in the provision of essential neurosurgical care. Executive Summary of the Global Neurosurgery Initiative at the Program in Global Surgery and Social Change. J Neurosurg 2018;130(4):1055–64.

8. Gupta S, Gal ZT, Athni TS, et al. Mapping the global neurosurgery workforce. Part 1: Consultant neurosurgeon density. J Neurosurg 2024;1–9.

9. Hoffman C, Härtl R, Shlobin NA, et al. Future Directions for Global Clinical Neurosurgical Training: Challenges and Opportunities. World Neurosurg 2022;166:e404–18.

10. Fuller A, Tran T, Muhumuza M, et al. Building neurosurgical capacity in low and middle income countries. eNeurologicalSci 2016;3:1–6.

11. Haglund MM, Kiryabwire J, Parker S. Surgical capacity building in Uganda through twinning, technology, and training camps. World J Surg 2011;35(6): 1175–82.

12. Leidinger A, Extremera P, Kim EE, et al. The challenges and opportunities of global neurosurgery in East Africa: the Neurosurgery Education and Development model. Neurosurg Focus 2018;45(4):E8.

13. Fuller AT, Barkley A, Du R, et al. Global neurosurgery: a scoping review detailing the current state of international neurosurgical outreach. J Neurosurg 2020; 134(3):1316–24.

14. Christie S, Chahine T, Curry LA, et al. The Evolution of Trust Within a Global Health Partnership With the Private Sector: An Inductive Framework. Int J Health Pol Manag 2022;11(7):1140–7.

15. Neurosurgeon AANS. Project Shunt: Dr. Karin Muraszko's Global Legacy. AANS Neurosurgeon. Available at: https://aansneurosurgeon.org/feature/project-shunt-dr-karin-muraszkos-global-legacy/.

16. Bankole NDA, Ouahabi AE. Towards a collaborative-integrative model of education and training in neurosurgery in low and middle-income countries. Clin Neurol Neurosurg 2022;220:107376.

17. Servadei F, Rossini Z, Nicolosi F, et al. The Role of Neurosurgery in Countries with Limited Facilities: Facts and Challenges. World Neurosurg 2018;112: 315–21.

18. Ogunfolaji O, Omar K, Bukenya G, et al. Neurosurgery equipment donation in Africa: a scoping review. J Surgic Protoc Res Methodol 2023;2023(1): snac023.

19. Da HP, Yang G-Z, et al. Technologies for global health. Lancet 2012;380(9840):507–35.

20. Rehman AU, Ahmed A, Zaheer Z. International neurosurgery: The role for collaboration. Int J Med Pharm Res, 2023;4(1):15–24.

21. Haji FA, Lepard JR, Davis MC, et al. A model for global surgical training and capacity development: the Children's of Alabama–Viet Nam pediatric neurosurgery partnership. Childs Nerv Syst 2021;37(2): 627–36.

22. Ukachukwu AEK, Seas A, Petitt Z. Assessing the success and sustainability of global neurosurgery collaborations: systematic review and adaptation of the framework for assessment of international surgical success criteria. World Neurosurg 2022;167: 111–21.

23. Kanmounye US, Shlobin N, Robert JR, et al. Foundation for International Education in neurosurgery: The next half-century of service through education. J Global Neurosurgery 2021. https://doi.org/10.51437/jgns.v1i1.28.

24. Santos MM, Qureshi MM, Budohoski KP. The Growth of Neurosurgery in East Africa: Challenges. World Neurosurg 2018;113:425–35.

25. Almeida JP, Velásquez C, Karekezi C, et al. Global neurosurgery: models for international surgical education and collaboration at one university. Neurosurg Focus 2018;45(4):E5.

26. El Khamlichi A. The World Federation of Neurosurgical Societies Rabat Reference Center for Training African Neurosurgeons: an experience worthy of duplication. World Neurosurg 2014;81(2):234–9.

27. Karekezi C, El Khamlichi A. Takeoff of African Neurosurgery and the World Federation of Neurosurgical Societies Rabat Training Center Alumni. World Neurosurg 2019;126:576–80.

28. Karekezi C, El Khamlichi A, El Ouahabi A, et al. The impact of African-trained neurosurgeons on sub-Saharan Africa. Neurosurg Focus 2020;48(3):E4.

29. Lippa L, Kolias A. Meeting the need: capacity building and social responsibility in neurosurgery. Acta Neurochir 2020;162(5):983–4.

30. Dada OE, Bukenya GW, Konan L, et al. State of African Neurosurgical Education: An Analysis of Publicly Available Curricula. World Neurosurg 2022; 166:e808–14.

31. Negida A, Raslan AM. The global neurosurg research collaborative: a novel student-based model to expand global neurosurgery research. Front Surg 2021;8:721863.

32. Negida A, Raslan AM. Invitation to the GNS-I Study; a global evaluation of traumatic brain injury in low-, middle-, and high- income Countries. Adv J Emerg Med 2019;3(3).

33. Elobu AE, Kintu A, Galukande M. Evaluating international global health collaborations: perspectives from surgery and anesthesia trainees in Uganda. Surgery 2014;155(4):585–92.

34. Boyke AE, Shlobin NA, Sharma V, et al. Letter: Operationalizing Global Neurosurgery Research in Neurosurgical Journals. Neurosurgery 2021;89(3): E171–2.

35. Servadei F, Cannizzaro D, Thango N, et al. In Reply: Operationalizing Global Neurosurgery Research in Neurosurgical Journals. Neurosurgery 2022;90(6): e195–6.

36. Uche EO, Sundblom J, Iloabachie I, et al. Pilot application of Lecture-Panel-Discussion Model (LPDM) in global collaborative neurosurgical education: a novel training paradigm innovated by the Swedish African Neurosurgery Collaboration. Acta Neurochir 2022;164(4):967–72.

37. Beveridge M, Howard A, Burton K, et al. The Ptolemy project: a scalable model for delivering health information in Africa. BMJ 2003;327(7418): 790–3.

38. Richardson GE, Gillespie CS, Bandyopadhyay S, et al. Hosting an educational careers day within the virtual paradigm: The neurology and Neurosurgery Interest Group experience. Cureus 2022; 14(1):e21162.

39. Hoffman C, Hartl R, Shlobin NA. Future directions for global clinical neurosurgical training: Challenges and Opportunities. World Neurosurg 2022;166: 404–18.

40. Rodríguez-Mena R, Piquer-Martínez J, Llácer-Ortega JL, et al. The NED foundation experience: A model of global neurosurgery. Brain Spine 2023; 3:101741.

41. Rubinger L, Gazendam A, Ekhtiari S, et al. Maximizing virtual meetings and conferences: a review of best practices. Int Orthop 2020;44(8):1461–6.

42. Lepard JR, Akbari SHA, Haji F, et al. The initial experience of InterSurgeon: an online platform to facilitate global neurosurgical partnerships. Neurosurg Focus 2020;48(3):E15.

43. Maleknia P, Shlobin NA, Johnston JM Jr, et al. Establishing collaborations in global neurosurgery: The role of InterSurgeon. J Clin Neurosci 2022;100: 164–8.

44. Higginbotham G. Virtual Connections: Improving Global Neurosurgery Through Immersive Technologies. Front Surg 2021;8:629963.

45. Foundation, Barrow Neurological. Healthcare Philanthropy Supporting Neuroscience. Available at: https://www.supportbarrow.org/blog/healthcare-philanthropy-supporting-neuroscience/#:~:text=Barrow%20Neurological%20Foundation%20provides%20support,neurology%2C%20vascular%20neurology%2C%20and%20more.

46. Smith LGF, Chiocca EA, Zipfel GJ, et al. Neurosurgery Research and Education Foundation funding conversion to National Institutes of Health funding. J Neurosurg 2022;136(1):287–94.

47. Javeed S, Pugazenthi S, Huguenard AL, et al. Impact of Neurosurgery Research and Education Foundation awards on subsequent grant funding and career outcomes of neurosurgeon-scientists. J Neurosurg 2023;139(1):255–65.

48. Global Neurosurgery Initiative. Program in Global Surgery and Social Change. Available at: https://www.pgssc.org/gnsinitiative#:~:text=In%20response%20to%20the%20unmet,and%20advocacy%20with in%20global%20neurosurgery.

49. CNS Foundation Impact Report. CNS Foundation.

50. Rolle M, Nahed BV. Global Neurosurgery and the Congress of Neurological Surgeons: Collaboration, Innovation, and Opportunity to Improve Care, Education, and Access. JGNS 2021;1(1):60–1.

51. Grossman A, Appleby S, Reimers C. Venture philanthropy: Its evolution and its future. Harvard Business School 2013. Available at: https://www.avpn.asia/wp-content/uploads/2013/07/VP_Its_Evolution_and_Its_Future_6_13_13_copy.pdf.

52. Zusman EE, Heary RF, Stroink AR. Philanthropy funding for neurosurgery research and program development. Neurosurgery 2013. https://doi.org/10.1227/01.neu.0000429863.50018.f0.

53. Bordelon B. How a billionaire-backed network of AI advisers took over Washington. Politico. Available at: https://www.politico.com/news/2023/10/13/open-philanthropy-funding-ai-policy-00121362.

54. Stevenson M, Youde J. Public-private partnering as a modus operandi: Explaining the Gates Foundation's approach to global health governance. Global Publ Health 2021;16(3):401–14.

55. Singer ME, Hack D, Hanley D. The power of public–private partnership in medical technology innovation: Lessons from the development of FDA-cleared medical devices for assessment of concussion. J Clin Transl Sci 2022;6. https://doi.org/10.1017/cts.2022.373.

56. Liang KE, Bernstein I, Kato Y, et al. Enhancing neurosurgical education in low- and middle-income

countries: current methods and new advances. Neuro Med Chir 2016;56(11):709–15.

57. Saha S, Beach MC. Impact of physician race on patient decision-making and ratings of physicians: a randomized experiment using video vignettes. J Gen Intern Med 2020;35(4):1084–91.

58. Traylor AH, Schmittdiel JA, Uratsu CS, et al. Adherence to cardiovascular disease medications: does patient-provider race/ethnicity and language concordance matter? J Gen Intern Med 2010;25(11):1172–7.

59. Greenwood BN, Hardeman RR, Huang L, et al. Physician-patient racial concordance and disparities in birthing mortality for newborns. Proc Natl Acad Sci U S A 2020;117(35):21194–200.

60. Persky S, Kaphingst KA, Allen VC Jr, et al. Effects of patient-provider race concordance and smoking status on lung cancer risk perception accuracy among African-Americans. Ann Behav Med 2013; 45(3):308–17.

61. Ikwuegbuenyi C, Adegboyega G, Nyalundja AD, et al. Public awareness, knowledge of availability, and willingness to use neurosurgical care services in africa: a cross-sectional e-survey protocol. Int J Surg Protoc 2021;25(1):123–8.

62. Musoke D, Boynton P, Butler C, et al. Health seeking behaviour and challenges in utilising health facilities in Wakiso district, Uganda. Afr Health Sci 2014; 14(4):1046–55.

Nongovernmental Organizations in Global Neurosurgery
Foundation for International Education in Neurological Surgery and Solidarity Bridge

Joyce Koueik, MD, MS[a], Lars Meisner, MD[a], Brandon G. Rocque, MD, MS[b], Richard Moser, MD[c], Robert J. Dempsey, MD[a],*

KEYWORDS

- Global neurosurgery • NGO • FIENS • Solidarity Bridge • Education

KEY POINTS

- Global surgery is a well-recognized emerging health inequity.
- Nongovernmental organizations (NGOs) are the important assets in bridging the gap of health care disparities.
- Foundation for International Education in Neurological Surgery and Solidarity Bridge are NGOs that aim to provide sustainable neurosurgical care through education and training for low- and middle-income countries.

INTRODUCTION

In the 1940s, the World Health Organization (WHO) was founded in Geneva with the aim to promote health across the globe so that everyone, everywhere, can receive the highest level of cares.[1] Part of their workforce was developing the millennium goals and the sustainable development goals. These included but were not limited to sanitation and hygiene, clean drinking water, immunizations, women's health, and communicable disease.[2] To bridge the gap in medical and surgical health, nongovernmental organizations (NGOs) in addition to the WHO have taken the lead in addressing the health care disparities between high-income countries (HICs) and low-income or middle-income countries (LMICs). In contrast to the WHO, NGOs are organizations formed independent of governments that focus on environmental, humanitarian, and social issues on both a national or global level. These are nonprofit in nature and dependent on collaborations, donations, and volunteering.

Being focused on medical and transmissible diseases primarily, the surgical aspect of health was overlooked, and the immense disparity in surgical care became apparent between HICs and LMICs. In the early twenty-first century, inequities in access to global surgery were recognized as a key target for improvement.[3,4] Since then, efforts to expand capacity to meet surgical needs to LMIC are on the rise.[5–7]

Thus, over the past few decades, many NGOs have launched to address the vast surgical disparities across surgical specialties such as general,

[a] Department of Neurological Surgery, University of Wisconsin, 600 Highland Avenue, Madison, WI 53792, USA; [b] Division of Pediatric Neurosurgery, Department of Neurosurgery, Children's of Alabama, University of Alabama at Birmingham, 1600 7th Avenue South, Lowder 400, Birmingham, AL 35233, USA; [c] Department of Neurological Surgery, UMass Chan Medical School, 55 Lake Avenue North, Worcester, MA 01655, USA
* Corresponding author. Box 8660 Clinical Science Center, 600 Highland Avenue, Madison, WI 53792.
E-mail address: dempsey@neurosurgery.wisc.edu

Neurosurg Clin N Am 35 (2024) 475–480
https://doi.org/10.1016/j.nec.2024.05.009
1042-3680/24/© 2024 Elsevier Inc. All rights are reserved, including those for text and data mining, AI training, and similar technologies.

obstetric, reconstructive, orthopedic, and neurologic surgery.

Initially, addressing the surgical disparity involved the availability of specialty surgeons, anesthetists, and equipment from HICs to travel to LMICs to perform the procedure at hand. This required a team of health care providers to travel with equipment to LMIC and perform surgeries over several week periods. However, the sustainability and accountability of this intervention have been challenged as both HICs and LMICs are cognizant of the limitations of this strategy. Medical trips where the visiting surgeon performs all surgeries without teaching the skill, including perioperative management, may result in more harm than good because such trips never meet the massive need, they may diminish the local doctors in the eyes of the population and invariably deplete local resources.

The need for neurologic surgery care in LMIC was identified in the 1960s and incredible efforts have been in place since then. This article describes 2 nongovernmental, nonprofit organizations that aim to provide sustainable neurologic surgery education and training to LIMCs around the world. The first is the Foundation for International Education in Neurological Surgery (FIENS) and the second is Solidarity Bridge. These 2 organizations are distinct in that they have identified ways to develop self-sustaining neurologic surgery services in LMIC with early education and teaching of the local physicians and surgeons.

FOUNDATION FOR INTERNATIONAL EDUCATION IN NEUROSURGERY
History and Objective

In the 1960s, an ad hoc committee of members from each of the 5 major American neurosurgical societies in existence at that time made a recommendation for the establishment of a foundation to coordinate international neurosurgical educational efforts. The result of this recommendation, the FIENS, was incorporated in April 1969. FIENS original mission was severalfold to facilitate American neurosurgeons who wished to engage in humanitarian neurosurgical work in low-resource settings; help neurosurgeons from low-resource settings find training in the United States; and provide advice to sites that wished to develop a neurosurgical department and other related activities.[8] By 1999, FIENS had partnerships in place in Indonesia, Nepal, Ghana, Zimbabwe, Thailand, India, China, Honduras, and Peru.[9] In 2019, FIENS celebrated its 50th anniversary, continuing to work toward those original goals and evolving with the changing landscape of international neurosurgery.

FIENS strives to improve neurosurgical capacity and access around the world through several distinct efforts, including development of curricula and educational programs, traveling fellowships for neurosurgeons from low-resource settings, financial support for neurosurgical residents to complete training, and ongoing educational activities such as a Virtual Visiting Professor program and in-person neurosurgery boot camps.

Development of Neurosurgical Training Curriculum

FIENS has prioritized establishment of self-sustaining programs focused on neurosurgical education in LMICs. Using this model, the FIENS has fostered global neurosurgical care worldwide.[10] The development of neurosurgical practices serves not only to provide vital care to patients but also drives growth of supporting staff and specialties such as anesthesia, operating staff, postoperative nursing, and ancillary services.[11] In addition to supporting volunteers from HICs, FIENS has been instrumental in creating curricula and training programs for neurosurgery in places where none previously existed, beginning to address the well-documented need for neurosurgical care worldwide.[5]

The process through which a neurosurgery residency curriculum was developed in East Africa demonstrates how self-sustaining education may be achieved. The initial work in East Africa began with Dr Paul Young, who began traveling to Nairobi, Kenya during the early 2000s.[12] Partnering with Kenyan neurosurgeon, Dr Mahmood Qureshi, FIENS surgeons and local collaborators began to develop a plan for a regional neurosurgical training program spread across multiple nations. The CURE Hospital in Mbale, Uganda; Mulago Medical Complex in Kampala, Uganda; Muhimbili Hospital in Tanzania; and Black Lion Hospital in Addis Ababa, Ethiopia joined in the collaboration in 2003 and 2004. The coalition of neurosurgeons from Uganda, Kenya, Tanzania, and Ethiopia developed a training program plan, including rotations at each participating hospital. This was then presented to the College of Surgeons of Central, East, and Southern Africa (COSECSA) as the potential accrediting body. The COSECSA approved the curriculum, allowing for standardization and certification of neurosurgical residents in these countries.[13] The curriculum was developed with a task force of neurosurgeons in the region, with the support of FIENS, which then provided equipment, supplies, and mentorship until the training program was self-sustaining. The training program lasts for a total of 6 years, with 2 years spent in the trainee's home program, focusing on general surgery, orthopedics, trauma, and intensive care. Four additional years of neurosurgical training follow, including rotations at the various participating hospitals and some outside programs. Training programs continue to be developed and address growing challenges, such as limitations in functional, endovascular, and open vascular exposure for residents, building on the foundation of FIENS throughout the world.[14,15] Additionally, new technologies, such as digital training or mobile neuroendoscopic training, have expanded the reach of FIENS and other international neurosurgery organizations.[16,17] These educational models have been repeated in the establishment or support of ongoing neurosurgical training programs in LMICs in Asia, Central America, South America, and Africa over several decades.

Foundation for International Education in Neurological Surgery Neurosurgical Training

Traveling fellowships have played an important role since the early days of FIENS. As described in the published report on FIENS activities in 1988, traveling fellowships have been a way to enhance the training of surgeons from low-resource settings as they establish their practice. In the early decades, this was thought to ideally involve a surgeon who was finishing residency training locally, who would then spend 3 to 12 months as a fellow in a North American program. One major limitation to this model was funding. If they were eligible for employment and clinical work, fellows were compensated by host programs. However, it was often difficult to secure employment and therefore funding.

Since 2017, FIENS has made major efforts to facilitate fellowships for young neurosurgeons from low-resource settings through 2 training programs named after their primary donors.

Basset fellowship
The Basset fellowship provides funding for neurosurgical trainees who are in the late stages of training, or who have finished their training within the past 5 years. Fellows spend several months at an established program in HICs for the purpose of further developing their skills and knowledge. Training focuses on surgical technique, research, and administration, with specific foci determined by fellows and fellowship mentors. A primary goal of the Bassett fellows is to empower individuals to create academic programs in their home countries.

To date, 38 trainees have been awarded the Bassett fellowship and 32 have completed the program. These people have returned to their countries in Asia, Central and South America, and Africa where they have either established or expanded neurosurgical care in areas of need.

Clack fellowship
Building on the success of the Bassett fellowship and recognizing the presence of excellent neurosurgical training programs throughout the world, FIENS in 2019 established the Clack fellowship. Clack fellows are neurosurgical trainees from areas with few existing neurosurgical resources, who are training in an established program in their region of the world. For example, fellowship support might be available for a trainee from Zambia, a nation with limited availability of neurosurgery, who is training at a university neurosurgery program in South Africa but is unable to continue without further funding. The Clack fellowship funds are intended to provide support for living and training expenses of the resident, allowing them to complete their residency with the intention of returning to their home country or region, where there is need for expanded neurosurgical care. To date, there have been 14 Clack fellows approved and 12 have completed the program.

The successful completion of these fellowships involves ongoing continued education of the fellows by FIENS. As the fellows are established as attending neurosurgeons, they in turn become educators in the program. Establishing a graduate in an area of need is only possible through ongoing support from the NGOs and graduate surgical education programs such as visiting professors and on-site educations programs such as boot camps.

Visiting Professor Program

Beyond providing funding to individuals and organization for the development of training curricula, FIENS has created opportunities for international collaboration in education. The Virtual Visiting Professor program invites international neurosurgical leaders to share their knowledge with fellows and trainees throughout the world. Prior Bassett and Clack fellows and neurosurgeons with a history of FIENS involvement serve as local hosts in regions with developing neurosurgical programs. The local host advertises the program locally, particularly to neurosurgical trainees and medical students. A senior neurosurgeon then gives a lecture, using an online platform, follows by a period for discussion and case review. This program not only allows for detailed discussions regarding cases and overall neurosurgical care but also allows for development of mentor–mentee relationships for young trainees. The focus on surgeons who have received support as Bassett and Clack fellows encourages continued involvement of these surgeons with FIENS.

Neurosurgery Boot Camp

Since 2015, FIENS has organized and hosted international boot camps for hands-on training of residents and junior neurosurgeons.[14] These programs are modeled after the boot camp for neurosurgery interns that is required for US residents, using the curriculum developed by the Society of Neurologic Surgeons in 2010. International boot camps have been held in Bolivia, South Africa, Myanmar, Zimbabwe, Nigeria, Singapore, Chile, Kenya, and Vietnam. These events have been organized with the assistance of local physicians, societies, foundations, and training programs in HICs such as the Henry Ford health neurosurgical program. They include various neurosurgical lectures, skill stations, case discussions, models, and simulators. This exposes residents to current techniques and equipment within the field while giving them an opportunity to network with residents outside their own programs and countries.

Since its founding in 1969, FIENS has striven to be a central resource for surgeons in high-resource settings who wish to be involved with neurosurgical education in low-resource regions of the world. In its early decades, FIENS also worked to be a clearing house providing information to surgeons in low-resource settings who were trying to build neurosurgery programs. With the COSECSA neurosurgery residency program, FIENS was able to help local surgeons leverage strengths of multiple stakeholders to develop a successful training model. The ongoing Bassett and Clack fellowships are natural extensions of FIENS' early work, now with funding to provide direct support. Finally, the Virtual Visiting Professor program and boot camps serve to maintain and strengthen FIENS connection to partners who are doing the important work of providing neurosurgical care where it is sorely needed.

NEUROSURGERY AND NEUROLOGY INSTITUTE: A PROGRAM OF SOLIDARITY BRIDGE

History and Objective

Solidarity Bridge is a nongovernmental, nonprofit US organization aimed to support surgical programs in Bolivia and Paraguay, comprising general surgery, gynecologic surgery, cardiothoracic surgery, and neurosurgery. The Neurosurgery and Neurology Institute (NNI) was founded in 2006 as a partner to Solidarity Bridge to mediate collaborations between physicians in the United States, Bolivia, and Paraguay, in conjunction with the

ministries of health of each of Bolivia and Paraguay. The goal is to establish measurable and sustainable actions to provide access to safe, timely, and affordable neurologic and neurosurgical health care.[18] This effort has been successful in mobilizing resources and enhancing the educational and surgical skills of trainees. Since then, the NNI has established learning initiatives through partner surgeries, fellowships, group discussion, and specialty dyads in the form of virtual and in-person conferences.

Resource Mobilization

Disparities in neurosurgical health care included (1) resource availability and (2) expertise in delivering care. To address the disparities in health care resources such as equipment and instruments, the NNI has equipped 6 Bolivian and Paraguayan public hospitals with high-speed drills, operating microscopes, neuroendoscopes, spinal and cranial instrumentation devices, ultrasonic aspirators, and others. Since 2006, more than 50 health professionals from 28 institutions and 13 states have embarked on medical trips to assist and teach in 82 complex surgeries such as arteriovenous malformation resection and endoscopic skull base surgeries in 6 cities in Bolivia and Paraguay.

Development of a Neurosurgical Education and Training

Solidarity Bridge is also focused on providing trainees in Bolivia and Paraguay with high-level neurosurgical education. The first neurosurgery boot camp took place in Bolivia in 2015 where 24 neurosurgical residents from 5 countries: Bolivia, Chile, Peru, Ecuador, and Argentina participated. This boot camp took place in conjunction with multiple societies including but not limited to Solidarity Bridge and FIENS.[19] The boot camp was repeated in 2018 before being interrupted by the COVID-19 pandemic requiring innovative new solutions to these educational challenges.

The COVID pandemic caused neurosurgery to embrace new methods of education as the world embraced virtual communication platforms. A teaching dyad platform was established between the University of Wisconsin and NNI, a program of Solidarity Bridge with Bolivia and Paraguay. This program is phased, starting with an online series of lectures, and progressing into in-person workshops as well as academic and clinical interactions between neurosurgery residents in Bolivia and Paraguay and faculty and residents at the University of Wisconsin. The overarching goal is to enhance the neurosurgical training of Bolivian and

Paraguayan residents while providing them with continuing medical education credit. Despite the known disparity in resources in health care across the United States and Bolivia and Paraguay, this educational effort has been providing the participants with exposure to varied approaches to care. Educators and trainees alike are cognizant of these differences and thoroughly respect the disparities. The virtual teaching sessions occur virtually twice a month and include the topics of pediatric, spine, tumor, epilepsy, vascular, and trauma neurosurgery. The lectures are translated real time, and attendees are evaluated with mandatory questions that they answer before and after each of the teaching sessions. The program also includes case presentation sessions, in which the residents get the opportunity to present challenging surgical cases to expert neurosurgeons in the United States.

Additional initiatives in Bolivia and Paraguay through NNI include educational activities such as hands-on workshops that promote teaching to sustain local ability to treat neurosurgical conditions. These include workshops on neurotrauma management, stroke and cerebrovascular advancements and treatment, pediatric epilepsy, and endoscopic skull base surgery (**Fig. 1**). The first microsurgery hands-on course took place in Paraguay in the summer of 2023. This involved a trip from Dr Keles, a research fellow from the microsurgery laboratory at the University of Wisconsin to provide microscopes and suture material for the residents to practice the microsurgery technique (**Fig. 2**).[20] Over a hundred of Bolivian and Paraguayan health professional have received some sort of training.

In 2023, the National Stroke Center Agreement was signed with the Paraguayan Minister of Health, and the Sucre Neurotrauma Initiative was established in Sucre, Bolivia.

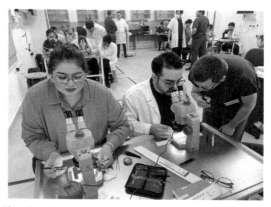

Fig. 2. Microsurgery hands-on course in Paraguay, June 2023. Dr Keles (in *blue* scrubs) teaching residents microneurosurgery.

Since its development, the NNI–Solidarity Bridge mission is to teach and train neurosurgical residents in Bolivia and Paraguay state-of-the-art neurosurgical procedures and techniques. This is done through collaboration with various institutes in the United States. These teaching opportunities are composed of in-person hands-on training session, in-person mentorship in complex surgeries, and virtual didactic lectures. Future direction includes establishing bidirectional exchange programs and scholarships for observer opportunities in the United States.

SUMMARY

The unique features of FIENS and NNI–Solidarity Bridge discussed in this article are their sole focus on establishing collaborations and teaching programs in LMIC to advance neurologic surgery and facilitate access to safe, affordable, and timely care. To guarantee that the endpoint of bridging the gap between developed and developing countries is sustainable, these organizations have emphasized the importance of helping the local physicians and neurosurgeons to optimize surgical care with the available resources at hand. Sustainability of the effort is key for continued improvement and long-term success.

DISCLOSURE

The authors have no disclosures.

REFERENCES

1. Brown TM, Cueto M, Fee E. [The transition from 'international' to 'global' public health and the World Health Organization]. Hist Cienc Saude Manguinhos 2006;13(3):623–47. A transicao de saude publica

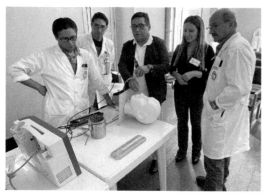

Fig. 1. Endoscopic skull base course in Sucre, Bolivia, November 2023.

'internacional' para 'global' e a Organizacao Mundial de Saude.

2. WHO. Millennium Development Goals (MDGs).

3. Dare AJ, Grimes CE, Gillies R, et al. Global surgery: defining an emerging global health field. Lancet 2014;384(9961):2245–7.

4. Meara JG, Hagander L, Leather AJM. Surgery and global health: a Lancet Commission. Lancet 2014; 383(9911):12–3.

5. Park KB, Johnson WD, Dempsey RJ. Global neurosurgery: the unmet need. World Neurosurg 2016; 88:32–5.

6. Shrime MG, Bickler SW, Alkire BC, et al. Global burden of surgical disease: an estimation from the provider perspective. Lancet Glob Health 2015; 3(Suppl 2):S8–9.

7. Meara JG, Leather AJ, Hagander L, et al. Global Surgery 2030: evidence and solutions for achieving health, welfare, and economic development. Lancet 2015;386(9993):569–624.

8. Mosberg WH Jr. Foundation for international education in neurological surgery, incorporated. J Neurosurg 1970;33(5):481–4.

9. Ablin G, Fairholm DJ, Kelly DF. Report of FIENS activities. Foundation for International Education in Neurological Surgery. J Neurosurg 1999;90(5): 986–7.

10. Bagan M. The Foundation for International Education in Neurological Surgery. World Neurosurg 2010;73(4):289.

11. Wright EJ, Nakaji P. Geopolitical forces and the challenges for developing world neurosurgery training. World Neurosurg 2017;101:750–1.

12. Dempsey KE, Qureshi MM, Ondoma SM, et al. Effect of geopolitical forces on neurosurgical training in sub-saharan Africa. World Neurosurg 2017;101: 196–202.

13. Leidinger A, Extremera P, Kim EE, et al. The challenges and opportunities of global neurosurgery in East Africa: the Neurosurgery Education and Development model. Neurosurg Focus 2018;45(4):E8.

14. Lepard JR, Corley J, Sankey EW, et al. Training Neurosurgeons in Myanmar and Surrounding Countries: The Resident Perspective. World Neurosurg 2020; 139:75–82.

15. Shah AH, Barthelemy E, Lafortune Y, et al. Bridging the gap: creating a self-sustaining neurosurgical residency program in Haiti. Neurosurg Focus 2018; 45(4):E4.

16. Nicolosi F, Rossini Z, Zaed I, et al. Neurosurgical digital teaching in low-middle income countries: beyond the frontiers of traditional education. Neurosurg Focus 2018;45(4):E17.

17. Piquer J, Qureshi MM, Young PH, et al. Neurosurgery Education and Development program to treat hydrocephalus and to develop neurosurgery in Africa using mobile neuroendoscopic training. J Neurosurg Pediatr 2015;15(6):552–9.

18. Souers C. A Bolivian medical mission experience. AORN J 2007;86(5):759–66.

19. Ament JD, Kim T, Gold-Markel J, et al. Planning and executing the neurosurgery boot camp: The Bolivia Experience. World Neurosurg 2017;104:407–10.

20. Keles A, Cancela AA, Moussalem CK, et al. A novel approach for free, affordable, and sustainable microsurgery laboratory training for low- and middle-income Countries: University of Wisconsin-Madison Microneurosurgery Laboratory Experience. Neurosurgery 2024. https://doi.org/10.1227/neu.0000000 000002814.

Engineering Principles and Bioengineering in Global Health

Joshua R. Harper, PhD[a,b],*, Steven J. Schiff, MD, PhD[c,d]

KEYWORDS

- Low-field MRI • Engineering in global health • Open source medical technology
- Sustainable health technology • Global health diagnostics

KEY POINTS

- A new paradigm for engineering of medical technology for low-resource settings is needed.
- Low-field MRI can provide useful diagnostic information in many settings where high-field MRI is neither feasible nor affordable.
- Machine learning algorithms are used to enhance the appearance of low-field MRI images, but caution is required because present versions can introduce structural artifacts that can affect clinical decision-making.

INTRODUCTION

Engineering has played an active role in medical practice since such practice was first recorded. The first known prosthetics were thought to be developed in the fifteenth century BC in ancient Egypt where an ancient mummy shows evidence of the replacement of an amputated toe with a prosthetic one.[1]

Industrialization has provided engineering solutions to medical problems at unprecedented depth and scale. The pharmaceutical industry alone is now worth an estimated US$1.4 trillion worldwide, while the global medical device industry was valued at over US$500 billion in 2023.[2] This enormous worth has, in some ways, made possible incredible advances such as clustered regularly interspaced short palindromic repeats (CRISPR), a genetic editing technology that promises to usher in a new era of personalized medicine in which technologies and therapies can be developed at the patient level.[3] Robotic-assisted surgery has become a common practice with at least 10 companies having already obtained Food and Drug Administration (FDA) approval.[4] Advanced use of machine learning and artificial intelligence has captured the imagination of researchers around the globe. Combined with the speed and affordability of modern computing, data can be assimilated, analyzed, and put into use in ways that were never before possible.[5] While these advances in technology are sure to reduce disability and death for many, this has not been the case for most.

In high-income countries (HIC), technological advancement in medicine is often a product of market-driving forces as much as it is medical need. Indeed, most health technologies are produced in HIC for high-income markets.[6] Much of the success of this sector has been driven by federal research funding. In the United States, National Institutes of Health funding was involved in every drug approved by the FDA from 2010 to 2016, totaling over US$200 billion in investment.[7] Without this enormous injection of high-risk funding, it is

a Facultad de Ciencias de la Ingeniería, Universidad Paraguayo Alemana, Lope de Vega nro. 1279, San Lorenzo, Paraguay; b Facultad de Informática, Universidad Comunera, Monseñor Bogarín 284, Asunción, Paraguay; c Department of Neurosurgery, Yale University, 333 Cedar Street, New Haven, CT 06510, USA; d Department of Epidemiology of Microbial Diseases, Yale University, 60 College Street, New Haven, CT 06510, USA
* Corresponding author. Universidad Comunera, Monseñor Bogarín 284, Asunción, Paraguay.
E-mail address: joshua.harper@ucom.edu.py

Neurosurg Clin N Am 35 (2024) 481–488
https://doi.org/10.1016/j.nec.2024.05.010
1042-3680/24/© 2024 Elsevier Inc. All rights are reserved, including those for text and data mining, AI training, and similar technologies.

unlikely that private investors would have funded the additional research and development (R&D) and clinical trials required to bring these products to market.

In low-and-middle income countries (LMIC), few resources exist for high-risk R&D focused on local problems, regardless of the market size. There are some examples of successful medical technologies developed by and for LMIC, such as Chhabra ventriculoperitoneal shunts for hydrocephalus,[8] but, in general, efforts have been inadequate and unfocused. There are excellent targeted funding mechanisms championed by HIC governments and organizations that expressly require the inclusion of LMIC researchers and entrepreneurs in the development phase of projects; however, these mechanisms often represent the health priorities of the HIC organization providing the funding and can be difficult to align with local governmental health care systems and policies. While important, these cannot substitute for the lack of local support and infrastructure to sustain development and incorporate new technology into health care.

Given the high cost of medical technology, many LMIC rely on donations from HIC governments or charitable organizations. Donations are an ineffective way to transfer technology from HIC to LMIC. A 2011 study estimated that between 40% and 80% of medical technologies donated to LMIC were in a state of dysfunction.[6,9] A recent 2019 study estimates that 50% of all donated radiographic technology in LMIC is nonfunctional.[10] It appears that despite the technological advancement of HIC medical devices, disappointingly little may have improved within the past decade in terms of global accessibility to critical devices.

The Lancet commission on Technologies for Global Health (2012) suggests that the development of frugal technologies should be prioritized to improve global access. They highlight 3 main barriers to the use of technology in global health: (1) the technology does not exist, (2) it exists but is not accessible, and (3) it exists and is accessible but is not adopted by the target health system.[6]

Following the 2015 report on Global Burden of Disease, Injuries, and Risk Factors, Barber and colleagues showed that there has been a global improvement in access to and quality of health care service related to so-called amenable deaths from 1990 to 2015. An amenable death is a death that could be avoided if current medical knowledge or technology were available and optimally applied at the time of care. Although improvement is encouraging, they also show that the pace of improvement has been significantly slower in LMIC, suggesting that the gap in treatment quality and access even for diseases we know how to treat is not sufficiently narrowing.[11] It is reasonable to conclude that the well-documented lack of access to technology faced by most of the population of the world plays a significant role in this avoidable loss of life.

While most investments in technology for health are focused on pushing scientific boundaries, engineering in global health, including HIC regions, faces an entirely different challenge. How do we provide universal access to the treatments and technologies that we already understand well?

In order to answer this basic question, engineers must understand priorities for greatest impact. Following the 2019 coronavirus disease pandemic, the importance of affordable and accessible diagnostics has risen to the forefront of global health. The 2021 Lancet commission on diagnostics identified diagnostic testing and diagnostic imaging as the largest gap in the care pathway for 5 of 6 considered conditions in a global study. In this study, 35% to 62% of patients in the care pathway who are screened for a disease do not pass to the diagnosis stage due to the lack of access to diagnostics. The study estimates that if this gap were reduced to 10%, disability adjusted life years lost to these conditions could be reduced by more than 38 million life years.[12] Presently, the commission estimates that 47% of the world has little or no access to diagnostics.

Availability of diagnostic testing is a crucial part of the care pathway. Treatments are often known, affordable, and achievable. In many cases, treatment can be as simple as prescribing the correct antimicrobial medication following identification of the infecting organism. Diagnostic imaging technologies, such as MRI, computed tomography (CT), and endoscopy, are those that are often crucial to care selection and are often lacking.

In the present article, we focus on the highly important role of diagnostic imaging in global health from an engineering perspective. We focus on 2 key challenges that can be met using engineering principles: (1) development of appropriate and sustainable technology and (2) reducing the need for expert interpretation of clinical results using machine learning methods. We develop these ideas by pointing out recent advances in the field of MRI and offering suggestions for future research.

LOW-FIELD MRI

MRI is one of the safest and most versatile diagnostic tools in modern medicine, but it is also one of the most costly. A commercial MRI scanner can cost around US$1 million per tesla of field strength,[13] not including the high cost of maintaining or building the specialized facility required to house it. Lower cost systems have recently been developed, which prioritize affordability and portability at the cost of image quality. However, there is rigorous and extensive evidence that the image quality from such systems is sufficient to guide clinical decision-making for certain diseases.[14] In terms of cost-to-benefit ratio for patients, it is likely that for diseases such as stroke, head trauma, and infant hydrocephalus, this technology will emerge as an effective option for diagnostic care in low-resource settings, and even in high-resource settings where the added benefit of point-of-care and radiation-free imaging may outweigh image quality decrement.

This is a critical concept in engineering for global health. Diagnostic technologies have historically been developed in high-resource settings for high-resource medical systems. As such, researchers and engineers have sought to maximize the data delivered by these devices. Yet, there is a cost of each incremental increase in information, and that marginal cost of additional information[15] is typically ignored in evaluating the additional benefit for patient outcome. Few studies have been performed to link advances in diagnostic data with superior clinical outcomes. There is an important distinction between data and information that we make here. Data may be sparse or vast but contain sufficient diagnostic information for a clinician to plan a proper course of treatment.

Commercially Available Low-Field MRI

The recently released 64 mT permanent magnet-based portable MRI system from Hyperfine, (Guilford, CT) has broken many use barriers in very little time. It is currently the only FDA-approved low-field system of its kind. Mazurek[16] demonstrated one of the first use cases in adult head imaging. The Hyperfine system was used to investigate stroke comparatively with CT and 1.5 T MRI systems. It was shown that the 64 mT system had a comparable diagnostic accuracy as compared to CT and 1.5 T systems; however, small bleeds in the brain remained undetected in some cases by the low-field system. The group extended this study by showing a detailed comparison between the low-field Hyperfine scanner and the gold standard in stroke care, CT, in a patient group of 177 who presented at the Yale New Haven Hospital with stroke symptoms. Sensitivity and specificity to intracerebral hemorrhage (ICH) was calculated to be 96%.[17] This number was an improvement over the initial study, which showed sensitivity and specificity of only 80% to small ICH. This drastic improvement is likely a product of an updated deep learning-based postprocessing technique, which was employed in the later study.

Mobile MRI has also been explored with the 64 mT Hyperfine system.[18] The entire system was installed in a large cargo van, and MRI was performed outside the hospital setting. Image quality in the van was comparable to that in the hospital demonstrating the capacity of this technology to be used in a variety of settings. This same workflow has been performed with portable CT and is an important strategy for global health where mobility of patients is often hampered by road conditions and the cost of travel. Such traveling diagnostic centers could be extended to other types of technologies as long as proper consideration is placed in the appropriate design of the technology for portability.

Though the 64 mT Hyperfine system has demonstrated the clinical utility of lower quality brain imaging, it still potentially suffers from the same failures in global health that other medical technologies face. The costs, about US$500,000 to lease for 5 years, may still be out of reach for many health ministries in LMIC. This also reduces the cost/benefit to patients, especially considering the recent release of higher field systems (0.5 T) that require no cryogenic replacement and can be purchased for a similar price. The hyperfine system is portable on a hospital floor, but is not so portable that it could navigate an extremely uneven or sloping floor, and the weight of its fixed magnet may render it incompatible with elevators in certain settings.

Open-Source Imaging Initiative

The open-source imaging initiative (OSII), launched in 2016, was formed to address this problem of accessibility and cost related to MRI research and use. The goal of the initiative is to create an expert knowledge base that has a unified goal of making available open-source hardware and software related to MRI.[19] In 2023, the first head only open-source MRI scanner was presented at the 2022 International Society of Magnetic Resonance in Medicine workshop on low-field MRI, following successful prototype builds at the Leiden University Medical Center in Leiden, The Netherlands,[20] and the Mbarara University of Science and Technology in Mbarara, Uganda.[21]

The original description of the device by O'Reilly and colleagues[13] and subsequent publications detailing improvements in homogeneity of the main magnet,[22] gradient design,[23] and in vivo imaging[20,24] show its potential to achieve clinically relevant brain imaging at a very low cost.

Importantly, in 2022, the system was successfully reproduced in less than 2 weeks at the Mbarara University of Science and Technology in Mbarara,

Uganda.[21] This was achieved by prefabricating the majority of the modular components in the Netherlands, and shipping all that was required to build a system as a "kit" to the laboratory in Uganda. Then, in collaboration with local students and researchers, the components were assembled into a working low-field MRI system. Efforts are ongoing in Mbarara to further develop this project into a device that can be used in clinical applications. Following this project, there are recent efforts in Asuncion, Paraguay, to replicate the open-source imaging system using primarily local tools and components.

This is an important milestone for diagnostic imaging in global health. Though there are still unanswered questions surrounding the role of open-source imaging system in medical technology, this project demonstrates what is achievable through the free sharing of knowledge and information. Echoing the recent call from the Seventy-Sixth World Health Assembly to strengthen diagnostics capacity, where diagnostic imaging was particularly noted to be lacking in the "developing world,"[25] this is a technology which, by design, is affordable, portable, and transferable to the region of use—all necessary requirements for a sustainable solution.

Open-source architecture and technology does not obviate commercial development for dissemination, service, maintenance, and training. It also does not obviate meeting all local medical safety regulatory requirements. But shipping technologies that meet the regulatory requirements in HIC to LMIC is not only a requirement but also another factor in escalating costs. It also is a practice that prevents the LMIC development of the industrial infrastructure to produce its own effective technologies to meet its own local needs.

Other Low-Field Systems

While we have chosen to highlight the Hyperfine and OSII low-field MRI systems, there are several other important projects that have contributed extensively to the field and show substantial promise for future deployment. One such is an 80 mT brain-only scanner developed at the Martinos Center of Massachusetts General Hospital, (Charlestown, MA).[26] This system has a unique built-in readout gradient in one direction, reducing the need for high-powered gradient amplifiers to perform imagining. Field inhomogeneities and gradient nonlinearity make distortion-free imaging a challenge; however, it is likely that future research with machine learning can resolve these issues.

Another emerging low-field system is described in another study.[27] This brain imaging system has a 0.055 T "double pole" permanent homogeneous magnet and is similar in concept to the Hyperfine system. A deep learning-based electromagnetic interference canceling scheme is used to remove noise from the raw signal data, forgoing the use of external shielding. The use of 2 disc-shaped magnets also keeps the design open for patient comfort, unlike the cylindrical shell designs of the OSII system and the Martinos Center system. The system is capable of T1, T2, fluid-attenuated inversion recovery (FLAIR), and diffusion-weighted imaging and has impressive data showing the utility for diseases such as stroke and tumor detection.

IMAGE PROCESSING AND ENHANCEMENT WITH MACHINE LEARNING

The increased affordability of high-quality electronics is largely responsible for the recent success of affordable medical technology. Beyond the affordability of the hardware itself, cost-effective electronics have made computational power more affordable, opening the door for the widespread use of machine learning in nearly every sector of society. Low-field MRI is no exception.

Data collection in MRI is a constant trade-off between time required for image acquisition, image quality, and signal-to-noise ratio (SNR). Faster imaging sequences are far more valuable in the clinic, for uncooperative young children, and for organizational workflows, but often suffer from reduced SNR, contrast, or resolution. In low-field MRI, this problem is compounded by the intrinsically lower SNR that comes with lower field strength. Advanced reconstruction, segmentation, and enhancement techniques have been developed to improve image quality and interpretation, in no small part driven by these factors.

Conventional MRI sequences make elegant use of the Fourier transform to convert the phase and frequency of the signal in spatial frequency space to image space. Unlike other bioimaging methods such as CT or radiography where image contrast is quantitative, image interpretation in MRI is largely reliant upon knowledge of the specific tissue properties (called T1 and T2 signal relaxation times) at the particular field strength of the system and for the imaging sequence being used. Magnetic resonance fingerprinting (MRF) has been shown to be a reliable approach to quantitative MRI.[28] MRF is an extension of compressed sensing, where multiple independent signal evolutions are used to identify the unique chemical properties, or fingerprint, of distinct tissues. It has been shown to be as fast as traditional clinical imaging sequences and potentially more robust to noise and bias. Beyond the potential use in clinical practice, MRF and other quantitative MRI methods offer the important potential for collecting large libraries of MRI data that can be used to train machine learning networks.

Another important advancement in the use of machine learning in image reconstruction is called automated transform by manifold approximation (AUTOMAP). AUTOMAP uses a supervised deep learning methodology to transform raw signal in frequency space to image space instead of the standard method that relies on the Fourier transform.[29] This is a powerful tool, since it allows for the possibility of removing noise and image artifacts directly and during the reconstruction process. It also enables the utilization of less perfectly smooth magnetic field gradients (linear) required to use the Fourier transform, requiring only that the matching of the object components in the MRI machine can be mapped one-to-one with a unique location of the image space. The quantitative nature also opens the door to repositories of learning libraries that are not specific to a particular MRI system or imaging sequence, allowing for the transfer of learning from one image dataset to another, a task that is difficult with conventional MRI techniques. AUTOMAP has been successfully applied to low-field MRI as well, demonstrating the ability of deep learning-based image reconstruction techniques to improve upon the achievable SNR in images that have inherently low signal and high noise.[30]

Deep learning methods have also been applied to a 55 mT low-field MRI system to remove noise and enhance images during reconstruction.[27,31]

This shielding free system has produced remarkably high SNR images that appear to show high anatomic accuracy with matched high-field (3 T) scans; however, some errors are always present.

The error between machine learning-enhanced images and conventional "ground truth" images is a point of concern for clinical practice. In the treatment planning of infant hydrocephalus, which occurs congenitally or following brain hemorrhages in premature infants (HIC dominant) or postinfection (LMIC dominant), knowledge of brain and cerebrospinal fluid (CSF) volumes is key to understanding the condition of the patient before and after surgical intervention.[32] Recent study has shown that deep learning methods can segment brain from CSF in CT images of hydrocephalus[33,34] with remarkable volumetric accuracy. In the same study, information from a learning library was used to perform super resolution and improve the quality of low-SNR and low-resolution images.[34] Traditional image quality metrics (ie, the Dice score) show significant agreement between enhanced images and ground truth in most cases; however, in the same study, a panel

of experts considered small errors between the enhanced images and ground truth to be potentially treatment altering, and it was concluded that machine-learned enhancement could at times be risky in the application of hydrocephalus treatment planning.

We illustrate how some of these risks arise in machine learning for medical images. For example, in facial recognition, the image to be recognized is already in the machine learning database. A noisy low-resolution picture just needs to be matched with the library's ground truth images. But in medical image analysis, each patient can present new one-off structures that are not present in the existing database. This enables algorithms to hallucinate structures that are not actually present as the machine learning attempts to bring information from its library of data to enhance the current image. Consider this simple imaging experiment performed in our laboratory on a 4 mT low-field MRI system described in an earlier study.[35] We constructed simple geometric phantoms as seen in **Fig. 1**. We trained a deep learning network on a library of ideal perfect geometric shapes without noise representing the phantom shapes (squares, triangles, and circles) as described in an earlier study.[34] By varying the field strength of an additional (prepolarizing) field between 0 T (off), 25 mT, and 50 mT, we produced images with increasing improvement in signal-to-noise. Notice that when the prepolarizing field was turned off, there is maximal noise in the raw images. At higher prepolarizing field, the deep learning network is able to reproduce the correct image. But when the signal-to-noise is low (the prepolarizing field is off), the deep learning network overlays the shapes in its library and produces an image that could exist, but in fact, does not. It hallucinates when bringing the library information to handle noisy and uncertain parts of the images.

In an ealier study,[34] small errors in image enhancement of infant hydrocephalus images were deemed to be potentially treatment altering by the panel of experts. A common machine learning hallucination was smoothing out the boundary of the fluid-containing ventricles within the brain, suggesting a subtle structural change used by clinicians to indicate that the pressure within the brain is increasing and may require surgery. Nevertheless, the unenhanced noisier and low-resolution images could be acceptable for treatment planning in many of these same cases.

In recent findings of Man and colleagues,[31] other examples of structural deep learning hallucinations were readily seen in the deep learning-enhanced imagery.[36]

These examples point to the need for further improvement in machine learning algorithms to

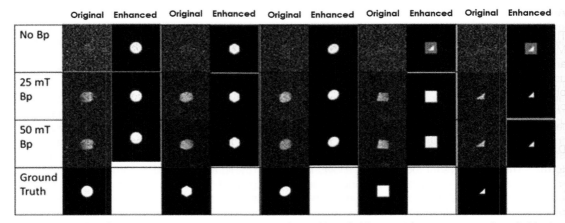

Fig. 1. The results of an imaging experiment on a prepolarized low-field MRI with a 4.23 mT readout field. Five geometric phantoms with cross sections of a circle, hexagon, oval, square, and triangle were constructed and filled with water. Images were collected with the prepolarizing magnetic field (Bp) off, at 25 mT, and 50 mT. Ground truth was synthetically generated using a computer. A deep learning library was trained with artificially degraded images at the SNR levels calculated from the experimental images. Enhanced images are displayed in each column next to the experimental images for comparison. Note the production of hallucinations in the images at upper right.

preserve structural fidelity. At present, there may be a need for a cultural shift in the acceptability of noisy images by clinicians from low-field MRI, until the rapidly advancing state of the art of machine-learned image enhancement enables more reliable anatomic fidelity. Presently, caution is required when applying machine learning techniques to enhance clinical data, and there is a need to show that enhancement adds clinical value beyond the risk of its use.

SUMMARY

The important role of the engineering of diagnostic technology in the health care pathway has gained increased attention. Simultaneously, the emergence of high-powered computing and machine learning in medicine means that the way we use diagnostic tools may be shifting. A diagnostic tool, such as an MRI scan of the brain, genetic screening, or even a simple blood test, is designed to deliver information in the form of data to clinicians to improve treatment specificity and patient outcome. Conventional technology has relied on the collection of high-quality, patient-specific data, which must be interpreted by an expert to generate a diagnosis. Yet the amount and quality of data required to improve patient outcome from a particular disease is often unclear. This uncertainty means that we have lacked an important component needed for global health engineering design—the ratio of outcome improvement to cost, and the incremental improvement from incremental increases in cost. These concepts have

long been embraced in the pharmaceutical industry, and we posit that developing such standards would be transformative for sustainable health engineering of medical devices.

The use of machine learning in health care enables a shift in the way we will look at diagnostic technology in the future. First, how much information is actually required to accurately diagnose a patient? This may allow for a significant reduction in the costs associated with producing a technology. Second, what are the potential roles for machine learning to improve the diagnostic accuracy of lower quality diagnostic tests? We have explored the lower limits of diagnostic usability for medical decision-making from lower quality image data, but defining the relationship of outcome improvement to cost and the incremental cost of improving data quality are fundamental properties that will be critical to improve the impact of medical technology on global health.

CLINICS CARE POINTS

- In global health, lower quality information may often be better than no information.
- Lower quality MRI images have been shown to be useful for many clinical diagnostic needs.
- Machine learning is fallible, and clinical integration should be cautiously pursued.

ACKNOWLEDGMENTS

The authors are extremely grateful to Dr Vishal Monga and Dr Venkat Cherukuri for developing and implementing the deep learning algorithms used in the illustrative experiment with geometric phantom imaging in this study, as well as the ongoing discussion surrounding the appropriate use of machine learning in medical diagnostics.

DISCLOSURE

Supported by NIH, United States R01HD085853 (S.J. Schiff, J.R. Harper), NIH Director's Transformative Award R01AI145057 (S.J. Schiff), R01HD096693 (S.J. Schiff), U01NS107486 (S.J. Schiff), an Equipment Transfer Agreement between Hyperfine and Yale University.

REFERENCES

1. Thurston AJ. Paré and prosthetics: the early history of artificial limbs. ANZ J Surg 2007;77:1114–9.
2. Mikulic M. "Global pharmaceutical industry–statistics & facts." Statista. 2024. Available at: https://www.statista.com/topics/1764/global-pharmaceutical-industry/#topicOverview. Accessed January 10, 2024.
3. Wang JY, Doudna JA. CRISPR technology: A decade of genome editing is only the beginning. Science 2023;379:eadd8643.
4. Peters BS, Armijo PR, Krause C, et al. Review of emerging surgical robotic technology. Surg Endosc 2018;32:1636–55.
5. Hamet P, Tremblay J. Artificial intelligence in medicine. Metabolism 2017;69S:S36–40.
6. Howitt P, Darzi A, Yang G-Z, et al. Technologies for global health. Lancet 2012;380:507–35.
7. Cleary EG, Beierlein JM, Khanuja NS, et al. Contribution of NIH funding to new drug approvals 2010–2016. Proc Natl Acad Sci USA 2018;115:2329–34.
8. Chhabra DK. The saga of the "Chhabra" shunt. Neurol India 2019;67:635–8.
9. Perry L, Malkin R. Effectiveness of medical equipment donations to improve health systems: how much medical equipment is broken in the developing world? Med Biol Eng Comput 2011;49:719–22.
10. Malkin R, Teninty B. Medical imaging in global public health: donation, procurement, installation, and maintenance. In: Mollura DJ, Culp MP, Lungren MP, editors. Radiology in global health: strategies, implementation, and applications. Cham (Switzerland): Springer International Publishing; 2019. p. 77–83.
11. Barber RM, Fullman N, Sorensen RJD, et al. Healthcare Access and Quality Index based on mortality from causes amenable to personal health care in 195 countries and territories, 1990–2015: a novel analysis from the Global Burden of Disease Study 2015. Lancet 2017. https://doi.org/10.1016/S0140-6736(17)30818-8.
12. Fleming KA, Horton S, Wilson ML, et al. The Lancet Commission on diagnostics: transforming access to diagnostics. Lancet 2021;398:1997–2050.
13. O'Reilly T, Teeuwisse WM, Webb AG. Three-dimensional MRI in a homogenous 27 cm diameter bore Halbach array magnet. J Magn Reson 2019;307:106578.
14. Kimberly WT, Sorby-Adams AJ, Webb AG, et al. Brain imaging with portable low-field MRI. Nat Rev Bioeng 2023;1:617–30.
15. Jackson CH, Baio G, Heath A, et al. Value of Information Analysis in Models to Inform Health Policy. Annu Rev Stat Appl 2022;9:95–118.
16. Mazurek MH, Cahn BA, Yuen MM, et al. Portable, bedside, low-field magnetic resonance imaging for evaluation of intracerebral hemorrhage. Nat Commun 2021;12:5119.
17. Mazurek MH, Parasuram NR, Peng TJ, et al. Detection of Intracerebral Hemorrhage Using Low-Field, Portable Magnetic Resonance Imaging in Patients With Stroke. Stroke 2023;54:2832–41.
18. Deoni SCL, Medeiros P, Deoni AT, et al. Development of a mobile low-field MRI scanner. Sci Rep 2022;12:5690.
19. Winter L, Periquito J, Kolbitsch C, et al. Open-source magnetic resonance imaging: Improving access, science, and education through global collaboration. NMR Biomed 2023;e5052.
20. O'Reilly T, Teeuwisse WM, de Gans D, et al. In vivo 3D brain and extremity MRI at 50 mT using a permanent magnet Halbach array. Magn Reson Med 2021;85:495–505.
21. Muhumuza I, Teeuwisse W, Harper J. On-site construction of a point-of-care low-field MRI system in Africa. NMR Biomed 2023. https://doi.org/10.1002/nbm.4917.
22. Tewari S, O'Reilly T, Webb A. Improving the field homogeneity of fixed- and variable-diameter discrete Halbach magnet arrays for MRI via optimization of the angular magnetization distribution. J Magn Reson 2021;324:106923.
23. De Vos B, Fuchs P, O'Reilly T, et al. Gradient coil design and realization for a Halbach-based MRI system. IEEE Trans Magn 2020;56(3):1–8.
24. O'Reilly T, Webb AG. In vivo T1 and T2 relaxation time maps of brain tissue, skeletal muscle, and lipid measured in healthy volunteers at 50 mT. Magn Reson Med 2022;87:884–95.
25. World Health Organization. First WHO model list of essential in vitro diagnostics: volume 1017. Genève, Switzerland: World Health Organization; 2019.
26. Cooley CZ, McDaniel PC, Stockmann JP, et al. A portable scanner for magnetic resonance imaging of the brain. Nat Biomed Eng 2021;5:229–39.

27. Liu Y, Leong ATL, Zhao Y, et al. A low-cost and shielding-free ultra-low-field brain MRI scanner. Nat Commun 2021;12:7238.

28. Ma D, Gulani V, Seiberlich N, et al. Magnetic resonance fingerprinting. Nature 2013;495:187–92.

29. Zhu B, Liu JZ, Cauley SF, et al. Image reconstruction by domain-transform manifold learning. Nature 2018;555:487–92.

30. Koonjoo N, Zhu B, Bagnall GC, et al. Boosting the signal-to-noise of low-field MRI with deep learning image reconstruction. Sci Rep 2021;11:8248.

31. Man C, Lau V, Su S, et al. Deep learning enabled fast 3D brain MRI at 0.055 tesla. Sci Adv 2023;9:eadi9327.

32. Kulkarni AV, Schiff SJ, Mbabazi-Kabachelor E, et al. Endoscopic Treatment versus Shunting for Infant Hydrocephalus in Uganda. N Engl J Med 2017;377:2456–64.

33. Cherukuri V, Guo T, Schiff SJ, et al. Deep MR Brain Image Super-Resolution Using Spatio-Structural Priors. IEEE Trans Image Process 2019. https://doi.org/10.1109/TIP.2019.2942510.

34. Harper JR, Cherukuri V, O'Reilly T, et al. Assessing the utility of low resolution brain imaging: treatment of infant hydrocephalus. Neuroimage Clin 2021;32:102896.

35. Obungoloch J, Harper JR, Consevage S, et al. Design of a sustainable prepolarizing magnetic resonance imaging system for infant hydrocephalus. Magma 2018;31:665–76.

36. Johnson PM, Lui YW. The deep route to low-field MRI with high potential. Nature 2023;623:700–1.

Global Partnerships in Neurosurgery
Mapping the Need

Saksham Gupta, MD, MPH[a,b,]*, Martina Gonzalez Gomez, MD, MSc[c], James M. Johnston, MD[c], Kee B. Park, MD, MPH[a]

KEYWORDS

- Global neurosurgery • Education • Workforce • Capacity • High-income country
- Low- and middle-income country

KEY POINTS

- The legacy of collaborative global neurosurgery partnerships between high-income and low-to-middle income countries (LMICs) has helped improve the quality of neurosurgery care and training worldwide.
- Partnerships between LMICs will have a growing importance to global neurosurgery.
- Delivering care in low-income countries remains a pertinent challenge that new educational models and policy may help solve.

INTRODUCTION

There are approximately 5 billion people who lack access to safe, affordable, and timely surgical care worldwide every year.[1] Low-and-middle income countries (LMICs) stand to lose nearly 0.5% of their annual gross domestic product from insufficient capacity every year, yet there are over 5 million LMIC patients who need, but cannot access, a neurosurgery operation annually.[2,3] A fully functioning health system depends on neurosurgery, particularly given the growing global burden of diseases such as traumatic brain injury, ischemic stroke, and epilepsy.[4] The burgeoning field of global neurosurgery has sought to remedy these deficiencies through clinical care, education, technological innovation, research, and policy.

Global neurosurgery, defined as "the clinical and public health practice of neurosurgery with the primary purpose of ensuring timely, safe, and affordable neurosurgical care to all who need it," has evolved drastically over the decades. While many early efforts consisted of intermittent mission trips without a structure in place to affect change, there has been a trend in developing sustained partnerships instead. Many of these sustained partnerships are between institutions or societies in high-income countries (HICs) and individuals or institutions in low-and-middle income country (LMICs), and most of them are directed toward long-term capacity building of the local workforce.

In this narrative review, consolidate evidence on the global neurosurgery workforce and the distribution of global neurosurgery collaborative partnerships between HICs and LMICs. Second, we aim to characterize the increasingly important contribution of partnerships between LMICs, the so-called "south–south" collaborations. After synthesizing these topics, we discuss how novel educational methods and policy contributions may help shape the international partnerships of the future.

---

[a] Program for Global Surgery and Social Change, Department of Global Health and Social Medicine, Harvard Medical School, Boston, MA, USA; [b] Department of Neurosurgery, Brigham and Women's Hospital, Boston, MA, USA; [c] Department of Neurosurgery, Division of Pediatric Neurosurgery, Children's of Alabama, University of Alabama at Birmingham, Birmingham, AL, USA
* Corresponding author.
E-mail address: sgupta@bwh.harvard.edu

Neurosurg Clin N Am 35 (2024) 489–498
https://doi.org/10.1016/j.nec.2024.05.011
1042-3680/24/© 2024 Elsevier Inc. All rights are reserved, including those for text and data mining, AI training, and similar technologies.

GLOBAL NEUROSURGERY WORKFORCE AND TRENDS

One of the goals of global neurosurgery is to develop and help sustain a sufficient neurosurgery workforce in each country. This includes general and subspecialist neurosurgeons, as well as several additional staff and medical subspecialists, including neurologists, intensivists, anesthesiologists, neuropathologists, neuroradiologists, intraoperative neurophysiologists, nurses, rehabilitation specialists, and bioengineers. Although neurosurgery services are known to be cost-efficient once they have been established, the upfront cost of creating a well-staffed and well-rounded neurosurgery service can be daunting.

Trends in the Neurosurgery Workforce

The World Health Organization (WHO) attempted the first comprehensive quantification of the neurosurgeon workforce in 2000, estimating there was 1 neurosurgeon for every 230,000 people in the world (~26,700 neurosurgeons according to the 2000 population census). A 2016 mixed methods report estimated there were 49,940 neurosurgeons, with the most rapid growth since 2000 occurring in Southeast Asia.[5] The most recent 2022 estimate of the workforce is 72,967 neurosurgeons worldwide, representing a worldwide pooled density of approximately 1 neurosurgeon for every 107,500 people (**Fig. 1**).[6] Despite this tremendous growth, there are still 29 countries and several more territories without a neurosurgeon, representing a population of 35 million people with no neurosurgeon in their borders.

The world is creeping toward the global neurosurgery workforce density of 1 neurosurgeon per 100,000 people, a conservative goal of how many neurosurgeons are needed, but wide disparities still remain in access to care.[7] The Western Pacific region has a nearly 15 times higher density than Africa (1.58 vs 0.11 neurosurgeons per 100,000 people). HICs overall have a nearly 20 times higher density than low-income countries (LICs; 2.44 vs 0.12 neurosurgeons per 100,000 people; **Fig. 2**). The annual rates of growth between 2016 and 2022 were highest in lower middle-income country (LoMICs) (26.0%) and upper middle income country (UpMICs) (21.3%). The rate of growth has been the most sluggish in Africa, but there have been 19 countries that doubled their overall workforce between 2016 and 2022, suggesting the potential for more rapid expansion in the near future.[6,8]

Recent studies have also estimated that the ideal ratio should be closer to 1 neurosurgeon per 65,000 people, if not even smaller, due to the rising breadth of neurosurgical diseases and the rising incidence of spinal stenosis, ischemic stroke, brain tumors, epilepsy, and so on.[7] It is well established that better access to neurosurgery means better population health, but the ideal "golden ratio" of neurosurgeons remains unknown. Each country likely has its own specific neurosurgery needs that dictate the amount and the ideal training of neurosurgeons for that population.

Should We Reconsider the "Neurosurgery Workforce"?

The global neurosurgeon workforce is a rudimentary global neurosurgery metrics, akin to quantifying overall mortality for brain metastases without

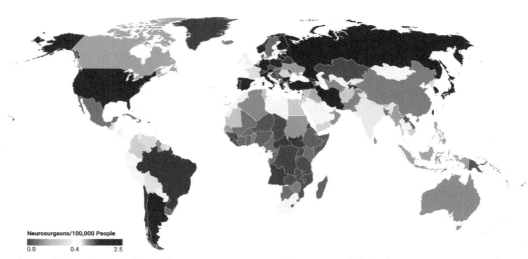

Neurosurgeons/100,000 People

0.0   0.4   2.5

Fig. 1. The workforce density of consultant neurosurgeons is demonstrated. (This figure was created with Datawrapper (Datawrapper GmbH).

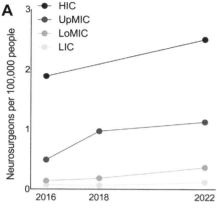

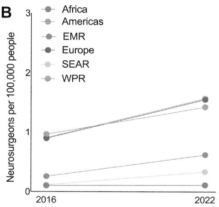

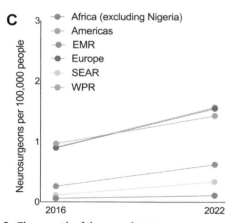

Fig. 2. The growth of the consultant neurosurgery workforce between 2016 and 2022 is demonstrated, stratified by World Bank income level (*A*), WHO region (*B*), and WHO region excluding Nigeria given potentially inaccurate estimates (*C*). (Gupta, S. et al., on behalf of the WFNS Global Neurosurgery Committee, EANS Global and Humanitarian Neurosurgery Committee, and CAANS Executive Leadership Committee. (2024). Mapping the global neurosurgery workforce. Part 1: Consultant neurosurgeon density. Journal of Neurosurgery, 141(1), 1-9. https://doi.org/10.3171/2023.9.JNS231615. An Open Access or Creative Commons publishing model conveys no rights to use this material in any format without written permission from the JNS Publishing Group.)

considering any oncologic factors, functional outcome, or overall patient well-being. This measurement alone is necessary, but not sufficient to understand strengths and gaps in neurosurgery coverage. However, mapping the consultant workforce helps identify regional workforce deficiencies, establish new regional referral pathways, and identify key regional thought leaders (particularly in LMICs) who can help move global neurosurgery forward.

Of note, there have been no comprehensive surveys to estimate the global workforce of neurosurgery nurses or other specialists that are critical to the delivery of neurosurgery. There are several nations that depend on general surgeons to perform basic, life-saving neurosurgery procedures as well, and quantifying these professionals may provide a more comprehensive and nuanced view of how neurosurgery gets delivered worldwide. Neurosurgery trainees are also a critical part of the workforce, often providing around-the-clock coverage for basic neurosurgery and neurointensive care in hospitals. There is an estimated pooled global trainee density of 0.14 neurosurgery trainees per 100,000 people.[9] The trainee density is considerably higher in HICs than LMICs, but it remains unknown what the ideal number of trainees should be to sustain a nation's workforce, and whether there is a "golden ratio" of consultants to trainees that can sustain a workforce.

A DEEPER DIVE INTO SUCCESSFUL, SUSTAINED HIGH-INCOME AND LOW- AND MIDDLE-INCOME COUNTRY COLLABORATIONS

There has been a rich tradition of HIC–LMIC collaboration in global neurosurgery. What started first as isolated mission trips, usually to provide clinical care in areas with virtually no neurosurgery capacity, has grown to more sustainable educational collaborations with long-term objectives. The phenomenon of neurosurgery departments or regional societies in HICs and LMICs partnering to provide bidirectional opportunities is known as "twinning" or a "dyad." Twinning has been a bedrock in global neurosurgery due to the long-term investment that these partnerships allow. It can help HIC trainees learn to manage more advanced disease with lower resources and help LMICs trainees gain exposure to subspecialty neurosurgery care and research methodology. Several neurosurgery faculty in LMICs maintain that twinning can be one of the most effective ways forward to bridge gaps in neurosurgery education.[10] Sustainable HIC–LMIC partnerships are almost universally appreciated by HIC and LMIC

Mapping Existing Partnerships

There have been several attempts to map, categorize, and quantify ongoing HIC–LMIC neurosurgery collaborations.[12,13] Traditionally, most HIC–LMIC partnerships have been between HICs in North America or Europe and LMICs in Africa, Latin America, and Asia.[14]

We applied the search methodology of the most modern HIC–LMIC global neurosurgery mapping attempt by Lu and colleagues, which searched for active partnerships up to February 2022, to expand the list of partnerships up to December 2024 (**Fig. 3**).[13] While capturing the total amount, scope, and intensiveness of different partnerships is beyond the purview of this narrative review, we identified several trends. Most HIC–LMIC partnerships are between HICs and middle-income countries (MICs) rather than LICs. The reasons for this are multifactorial: LICs are less likely to have any neurosurgeons to partner with, have less overall health care infrastructure and spending, and have more political instability that can destabilize partnerships.[15,16] There are notably fewer partnerships in West and Sub-Saharan Africa (see **Fig. 3**). There are also several MICs in Central Asia, Central America, and South America with no HIC–LMIC partnerships.

Maps like these are helpful in documenting global neurosurgery partnerships and progress, but do not provide the full picture of what is needed for neurosurgery services to thrive. For instance, they do not include the equipment available to neurosurgeons in LMICs. International subspecialty neurosurgery groups such as North American Skull Base Society and Mission Thrombectomy 2020+ can utilize their expertise to study specialty-specific problems and develop plans to improve subspecialty neurosurgery capacity in LMICs, including the technology and equipment needed to perform each case safely.

Maps may also be made into real-time, usable vehicles to simultaneously understand the state of global neurosurgery partnerships and learn how to get involved. InterSurgeon serves as a premier model to do this by fostering connections within the global surgery community to advance clinical care, teaching, training, research, and the provision and maintenance of surgical equipment.[17,18] Its matching algorithm helps individuals and institutions identify potential partnership opportunities and gaps in service delivery. InterSurgeon's reach has also expanded significantly through collaborations with global surgery advocacy organizations such as the G4 Alliance.

In the following sections, we highlight examples of two of the most common types of HIC–LMIC partnerships, organizational partnerships backed by neurosurgery societies, and bi-institutional partnerships between two individual neurosurgery departments.

Organizational Partnerships

Large global neurosurgery organizations have played a major part in promoting HIC–LMIC partnerships. These organizations include the Foundation for International Education in Neurological Surgery (FIENS), Neurosurgery Education and Development Foundation (NEDF), Mission Brain, and others. These organizations facilitate involvement by interested neurosurgeons by helping obtain funding, providing an infrastructure for

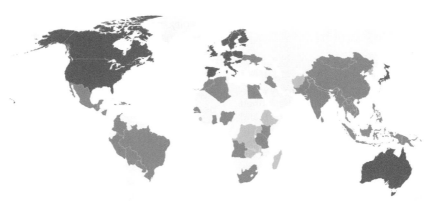

Fig. 3. Building on previous studies, a distribution of high-/middle-/low-income country actors who are a part of at least one HIC–LMIC partnership is displayed (*blue*, high-income country partner; *dark green*, middle-income country partner; *light green*, low-income country partner).[12,13]

involvement, and developing long-standing relationships with LMIC institutions. They open an avenue for all neurosurgeons to participate. Indeed, a survey of over 70 pediatric neurosurgeons involved in HIC–LMIC partnerships found that while most neurosurgeons worked through an existing organization (most commonly, CURE Uganda, FIENS, and the World Pediatric Project).[19]

FIENS has been one of the standard bearers in developing sustainable collaborative educational models between HICs and LMICs. The organization has emphasized "service through education" through its existence from 1969 to the present day, though it has changed its approach away from service delivery through mission trips to a health system strengthening approach by bolstering the local neurosurgery workforce and health sector. FIENS has organized several twinning programs, including Myanmar—Henry Ford and Bolivia—Solidarity Bridge Initiative partnerships and has organized several neurosurgery trainee education boot camps.[10,20,21] The organization has also prevented "brain drain" of the LMIC neurosurgeons by providing equipment and infrastructure support, as well as continuing education opportunities to its network of trainees.[22]

The NEDF started in 2006 as an organization to teach endoscopy for pediatric neurosurgery in Sub-Saharan Africa. It has developed a long-term, existing partnership with the Tanzanian Mnazi Mmoja Hospital. HIC members of this partnership have explored the casemix, local expertise, and infrastructure available in the region while helping provide clinical care and education to build local expertise. By 2014, the NEDF was able to partner with the ministry of health in Tanzania to create the Mnazi Mmoja NEDF Institute, a comprehensive clinical and education center. This partnership has involved hundreds of volunteer surgeons from HICs.[23] Over 25,000 patients have been evaluated and nearly 2000 operations have been performed or taught through this organization. The institute has supported over 15 scholarships and educational courses for Tanzanian neurosurgeons and nurses.[24]

There have been several HIC organizations from the United States, Canada, Spain, and Luxembourg that have contributed to clinical care and education in Peru. One example of a long-standing collaboration is between International Neurosurgical Children's Association (INCA) and the hospital Maria Auxiliadora in Lima Peru. After over 15 years of partnerships for clinical education, this site has become an independent neuroendoscopy training center for pediatric neurosurgery applications to the point where all of their residents receive training in neuroendoscopy.[25,26]

Bi-institutional Partnerships

The benefits of these "twinning" or "dyad" programs include bidirectional trainee transfers more easily, streamlined communication, and more specific and targeted goals. They may also facilitate fellowships for LMIC trainees in HICs, which can teach LMIC neurosurgeons how to apply various technologies for patient care. Although this training is not in their local context, it can guide what LMIC neurosurgeons advocate for, such as the multimodal Malaysian image-guided neurosurgery operating suite designed by several Malaysian neurosurgeons who had completed fellowship in an HIC.[27]

The majority of dyads have been with countries in Africa.[13] The Duke Global Neurosurgery and Neurology (DGNN) partnership with Mbarara Regional Referral Hospital and Mulago National Referral Hospital in Uganda has helped develop subspecialty neurosurgery care for over 15 years.[28] The DGNN dyad has also helped create the Ugandan neurosurgery training program at these locations. A long-standing collaboration between neurosurgeons at the Weill Cornell Medical Center and multiple institutions in Dar es Salaam, Tanzania, also demonstrates the capacity to transfer knowledge on specialized neurosurgery, including scoliosis surgery.[29] The CURE hospital in Uganda has developed into an international center of excellence for pediatric neuroendoscopic surgery, specializing in the combined endoscopic third ventriculostomy and choroid plexus cauterization operation for hydrocephalus developed there by Dr Benjamin Warf.[30] This center has also provided evidence for the efficacy of this operation, which has elevated the standard of care for pediatric hydrocephalus worldwide.[31]

Southeast Asia and the Western Pacific have been important regions of HIC–LMIC collaboration in global neurosurgery. Several countries in these regions have a growing number of neurosurgeons and have sought subspecialized education. The Alabama-Vietnam partnerships to teach subspecialty pediatric and epilepsy neurosurgery care have been long-term, sustainable partnerships that have provided advanced clinical training, out-of-country fellowship and opportunities training for ancillary staff who are necessary to build a service (ie, neurophysiologists).[32,33] Several LMIC and HIC neurosurgeons are faculty at an educational trainee boot camp in Myanmar.[34]

There are also examples of dyads in Eastern Europe. The copilot program, developed in conjunction with several US-based and Ukrainian neurosurgeons, was created to increase the complex case capacity of Ukrainian neurosurgeons.[35] Through this program, dozens of lectures have been given and dozens of highly complex cases have been performed by mixed Ukrainian/US teams.

The Caribbean islands in North America provide several additional challenges to establishing neurosurgery HIC–LMIC dyads. Several islands have no neurosurgery capacity aside and referrals to other islands for neurosurgery emergencies can take prohibitively long.[36,37] Despite attempts to form an HIC–LMIC partnership to create the first neurosurgery training program in Haiti, this program is now defunct, leaving only 5 neurosurgeons in the country to manage 12 million people according to a report by Haitian surgeons.[38] Consequently, there is a high degree of task-shifting in the region, with general surgeons performing a considerable amount of general neurosurgery cases.[37]

It is noteworthy that there are few partnerships with LICs specifically. Establishing educational relationships with LICs can prove challenging due to a lack of internal infrastructure, despite eager participants in HICs and LICs. In these nations, dyads that conduct mission trips to provide clinical care have been more common. A mission trip reported in Liberia involved heavy preplanning and a multidisciplinary team of volunteers and a Liberian neurosurgeon but was ultimately limited by infrastructure-related problems.[39] Somaliland has several external visiting surgeons performing basic neurosurgery procedures, but no permanent internal neurosurgeons.[40] HIC–LIC dyads can work with the general surgeons in a population and help them attain specialty neurosurgeon training. This has been the mode of operation in Sierra Leone, where several US-based neurosurgeons and the mission:brain organization have supported and funded efforts to train general surgeons at the WFNS Rabat training center, which was driven by Sierra Leonean health officials. A multilateral partnership between several HIC and MIC institutions to provide neurosurgery supplies and Afghanistan has progressed forward, but programs like this can be difficult to sustain in regions experiencing fraught political and humanitarian crises.[41] Mission trips in neurosurgery may have a mixed long-term effect because external aid is associated with a growth in the neurosurgery workforce, but also causes governments to spend less of their money on health care spending.[42] This may contribute to higher cost-sharing for patients which could make access to care difficult despite more neurosurgeons.

Ongoing barriers for high-income country/low-and-middle-income country partnership participation

The burgeoning interest of LMIC trainees presents an opportunity to bolster the future workforce with highly trained and subspecialized neurosurgeons, but they face barriers to participate in high-income country/low-and-middle-income country (HIC–LMIC) partnerships. Surveys of African trainees have consistently shown insufficient opportunities to attend venues where they could meet HIC partners and mentees, including research meetings, attend educational conferences, and access international cadaveric dissection courses.[43,44] Neurosurgeons and trainees in HICs also report high levels of enthusiasm to participate in global neurosurgery endeavors.[14,19] Barriers to joining have included obtaining a consistent funding source, interference with one's practice, interference with one's family or personal life, and identifying potential LMIC partners or organizations that can provide an infrastructure for participation.[11,14]

THE RECENT RISE OF PARTNERSHIP BETWEEN LOW-AND-MIDDLE INCOME COUNTRIES

There has been a recent wave of ground-up drive and excitement among LMIC neurosurgeons and trainees to identify their own needs and develop partnerships to meet them.[45,46] This has led to the rise of partnership between LMICs to support each other. While the topic of this article and the majority of the global neurosurgery literature on international partnerships have focused on HIC–LMIC partnership, there are increasing examples of these promising partnerships.

The WFNS training center in Rabat, Morocco, has been a fertile training ground for young African neurosurgeons from across the continent. This center is spearheaded by several prominent LMIC neurosurgeons and has graduated dozens of trainees, many of whom now practice in low-income country (LICs).[47] Decentralized training centers like those organized by the West African College of Surgeons and the College of Surgeons of East, Central, and Southern Africa (COSECSA) can also provide subspecialty surgical exposure to trainees in the region. Regional centers such as WFNS Rabat and COSECSA also provide a pipeline to bring training opportunities for medical graduates in countries where there are no training programs or neurosurgeons, including Sierra Leone among others.[48] An example of a smaller scale bi-institutional partnership between LMICs is the Angola–Brazil training experience, which has allowed an Angolan trainee to learn subspecialty neurosurgery in Brazil.[49]

There are several reports of arrangements where neurosurgeons from LMICs provide clinical coverage and training in countries, particularly LICs with few or no neurosurgeons. For instance, neurosurgeons from the United States, India, and Tajikistan have provided neurosurgery coverage and basic training in Somaliland, where there are no practicing neurosurgeons.[40] These trips help innumerable patients who otherwise may have no virtually no access to a neurosurgeon until a more permanent solution is developed by the government and external parties. It is likely that there are several of these arrangements that are not reported in the literature, particularly not in Western, English-based journals indexed in databases such as PubMed.

The next decade of progress in global neurosurgery is likely to involve more of these partnerships, which provide benefits that HIC–LMIC partnerships cannot. Focused collaboration between nearby LMICs can lead to the development of region-specific surgical techniques and preoperative/postoperative management protocols. Partnerships between neighboring countries may organically develop efficient and dependable international referral pathways for complex cases. Neighboring LMIC partners may find economic benefit by sharing expensive resources, such as 3 dimensional printers for implants and neuroangiography suites, rather than paying exorbitant costs for their population to be treated in distant HICs or relying on unpredictable foreign aid to temporarily fund services. Neurosurgery agreements between LMICs may serve as "medical diplomacy" with the hope that political agreements for noncontroversial issues such as neurosurgical care may ease communication about more contentious issues. These concepts should be considered as the role of HICs may begin to change in certain regions to help support, rather than lead, sustainable LMIC–LMIC dyads and collaborations.

TRENDS IN EDUCATION

Improving surgical education remains a top priority for global neurosurgery partnerships given the challenges that threaten the training pipeline in LMICs. Several countries have no trainees to maintain their consultant workforce, and the format of neurosurgery training varies widely in different contexts.[5,9] Trainees in LMICs are also more likely to have to pay for training rather than being afforded a salary or stipend.[50] There are several opportunities for educational innovation for HIC–LMIC partnerships, including the incorporation of novel technologies and subspecialty training.

Technological Advances in Education

The past decade has seen a wave of new digital and simulation technologies. A variety of virtual tools and simulation models may be effective tools to supplement education when cadaver laboratories are

unavailable.[45,51–53] These include UpSurgeOn simulation models, which can help trainees understand complex cranial approaches.[41,54] As the world has become more interconnected by teleconferencing platforms, there have also been shifts to expand global collaboration opportunities. With this rapid growth of new options, the Global Neurosurgery Education Summit served as an attempt to organize these new and disparate teaching modalities for global neurosurgery.[55]

Advanced Training

There is a growing recognition to foster subspecialty training given that trainees in some LMICs report having insufficient subspecialty case exposure to manage their population's needs.[9] While subspecialty neurosurgery can be expensive, some aspects of subspecialty training (such as how to perform a tailored preoperative workup, understand neuroanatomy within a difficult case, and monitor patients postoperatively) could be relatively cost-efficient. An international didactic course to discuss adapting the clinical approach for challenging neurosurgery cases in the Sub-Saharan Africa context spearheaded by Nigerian and Swedish neurosurgeons was found to be helpful to neurosurgeons.[56]

TRENDS IN POLICY

HIC–LMIC neurosurgery partnerships are becoming active in global health policy by forming coalitions, finding their political voice, and advocating for patients worldwide. Neurosurgeons in policy can address the specific needs of their health care systems and ensure the delivery of high-quality neurosurgical care. An active area for neurosurgery policy research is how to obtain sustained funding through health ministries. Neurosurgery procedures are highly cost-effective but can present a prohibitively high upfront cost for an LMIC ministry of health or a public hospital to afford. For example, fewer than 20% of LICs have a single comprehensive stroke center even though mechanical thrombectomy is one of the most clinically effective and cost-effective interventions in all of medicine.[57]

Global neurosurgery is still in its policy nascency but has already begun to make an impact. Neurosurgeons are helping shape National Surgical, Obstetric, and Anesthesia Plans (NSOAPs), which direct countries' long-term surgery plans and funding structures.[58] Furthermore, neurosurgeons within the Global Alliance for Prevention of spina bifida and the G4 Alliance worked together with a variety of stakeholders and members of civil society acting as the driving force of a resolution to prevent spina bifida and other neural tube defects through advocacy for implementation of folic acid food fortification. The resolution World Health Assembly (WHA) 76.19 was adopted at the 76th WHA in May 2023 under the umbrella of the United Nations Decade of Action on Nutrition (2016–2025).[59] Another opportunity for neurosurgeons to be involved in policy is the WHO Intersectoral Global Action Plan for Epilepsy and other neurological disorders 2022 to 2031 has provided a window for neurosurgeons to become involved with like-minded global neurologists in executing multidisciplinary policy.[60]

One complicating feature in policy is that different political bodies at different levels (ie, municipal, national, and international) have varying jurisdiction and funding to execute their policies. Policy crafted by certain global bodies may have an amplifying and aspirational effect (ie, the WHO), while policy by smaller bodies may be able to implement concrete change directly through funding and personnel support (ie, a national health ministry's NSOAP). It would be beneficial for neurosurgeons to open dialogues with public health and policy officials to determine the best way to push various elements of the global neurosurgery agenda forward.

SUMMARY

Collaboration and partnership have propelled the field of global neurosurgery forward. Initially driven by HIC–LMIC partnerships involving HIC actors from North America and Europe and LMIC actors from Africa, Latin America, and Asia, these partnerships have become more complex and interconnected, and there has been a rise in LMIC–LMIC partnerships. Additional challenges remain, including how to build sustainable partnerships in LICs specifically and how to modernize our approach to education and policy to meet the needs of neurosurgeons and patients.

CLINICS CARE POINTS

- HIC-LMIC partnerships provides bidirectional benefits to improve neurosurgery care.
- There is a growing trend of LMIC-LMIC partnerships that should be promoted.
- Innovative educational modalities provide a way to accelerate training or provide it in an area where it previously did not exist.
- Policy in global neurosurgery is in its nascency and has a growing role in supporting and funding partnerships.

REFERENCES

1. Meara JG, Leather AJM, Hagander L, et al. Global Surgery 2030: evidence and solutions for achieving health, welfare, and economic development. Lancet 2015;386(9993):569–624.
2. Dewan MC, Rattani A, Fieggen G, et al. Global neurosurgery: the current capacity and deficit in the provision of essential neurosurgical care. Executive Summary of the Global Neurosurgery Initiative at the Program in Global Surgery and Social Change. J Neurosurg 2018;1–10.
3. Rudolfson N, Dewan MC, Park KB, et al. The economic consequences of neurosurgical disease in low- and middle-income countries. J Neurosurg 2018;130(4). https://doi.org/10.3171/2017.12.JNS17281.
4. Dewan MC, Rattani A, Gupta S, et al. Estimating the global incidence of traumatic brain injury. J Neurosurg 2018;130(4). https://doi.org/10.3171/2017.10.JNS17352.
5. Mukhopadhyay S, Punchak M, Rattani A, et al. The global neurosurgical workforce: a mixed-methods assessment of density and growth. J Neurosurg 2019;130(4):1142–8.
6. Gupta S, Gal ZT, Athni TS, et al. Mapping the global neurosurgery workforce. Part 1: Consultant neurosurgeon density. J Neurosurg 2024;1(aop):1–9.
7. Rosman J, Slane S, Dery B, et al. Is there a shortage of neurosurgeons in the United States? Neurosurgery 2013;73(2):354–5 [discussion 365–6].
8. Uche EO, Ryttlefors M, Tisell M. Scaling up global collaborations for neurosurgical education and care capacity development in west africa: are there low-hanging fruits where it tolls? World Neurosurg 2020;139:512–8.
9. Gupta S, Gal ZT, Athni TS, et al. Mapping the global neurosurgery workforce. Part 2: Trainee density. J Neurosurg 2024;1(aop):1–7.
10. Lepard JR, Corley J, Sankey EW, et al. Training neurosurgeons in myanmar and surrounding countries: the resident perspective. World Neurosurg 2020;139:75–82.
11. Mediratta S, Lippa L, Venturini S, et al. Current state of global neurosurgery activity amongst European neurosurgeons. J Neurosurg Sci 2022. https://doi.org/10.23736/S0390-5616.21.05447-3.
12. Olivieri DJ, Baticulon RE, Labuschagne JJ, et al. Geospatial mapping of international neurosurgical partnerships and evaluation of extent of training and engagement. World Neurosurg 2020;144:e898–907.
13. Lu Z, Tshimbombu TN, Abu-Bonsrah N, et al. Transnational capacity building efforts in global neurosurgery: a review and analysis of their impact and determinants of success. World Neurosurg 2023. https://doi.org/10.1016/j.wneu.2023.01.120.
14. Nundy S, Kakar A, Bhutta ZA. How to practice academic medicine and publish from developing

countries? A practical guide. Singapore: Springer Nature; 2021.

15. Dirks M, Schmidt T. The relationship between political instability and economic growth in advanced economies: Empirical evidence from a panel VAR and a dynamic panel FE-IV analysis. Ruhr Economic Papers 2023. https://doi.org/10.4419/96973166. Published online.

16. Aisen A, Veiga FJ. How does political instability affect economic growth? IMF; 2011. Available at: https://www.imf.org/en/Publications/WP/Issues/2016/12/31/How-Does-Political-Instability-Affect-Economic-Growth-24570. [Accessed 13 January 2024].

17. Lepard JR, Akbari SHA, Haji F, et al. The initial experience of InterSurgeon: an online platform to facilitate global neurosurgical partnerships. Neurosurg Focus 2020;48(3). https://doi.org/10.3171/2019.12.FOCUS19859.

18. Maleknia P, Shlobin NA, Johnston JM Jr, et al. Establishing collaborations in global neurosurgery: The role of InterSurgeon. J Clin Neurosci 2022;100:164–8.

19. Davis MC, Rocque BG, Singhal A, et al. State of global pediatric neurosurgery outreach: survey by the International Education Subcommittee. J Neurosurg Pediatr 2017;20(2):204–10.

20. Kanmounye US, Shlobin NA, Robert JRJ, et al. Foundation for international education in neurosurgery: the next half-century of service through education. JGNS 2021;1(1):68–72.

21. Ament JD, Kim T, Gold-Markel J, et al. Planning and executing the neurosurgery boot camp: the bolivia experience. World Neurosurg 2017;104. https://doi.org/10.1016/j.wneu.2017.05.046.

22. Sedney CL, Siu J, Rosseau G, et al. International neurosurgical volunteerism: a temporal, geographic, and thematic analysis of foundation for international education in neurological surgery volunteer reports. World Neurosurg 2014;82(6):963–8.

23. Rodríguez-Mena R, Piquer-Martínez J, Llácer-Ortega JL, et al. The NED foundation experience: A model of global neurosurgery. Brain Spine 2023; 3:101741.

24. mnazi Mmoja Ned Surgical institute. nedfundacion.org. Available at: https://nedfundacion.org/projects/neurosurgery/mnazi/?lang=en. [Accessed 14 January 2024].

25. Bocanegra-Becerra JE, Castillo-Huerta NM, Ludeña-Esquivel A, et al. The humanitarian aid of neurosurgical missions in Peru: A chronicle and future perspectives. Surg Neurol Int 2022;13. https://doi.org/10.25259/SNI_940_2022.

26. Jandial R, Narang P, Brun JD, et al. Optimizing international neurosurgical outreach missions: 15-year appraisal of operative skill transfer in Lima, Peru. Surg Neurol Int 2021;12. https://doi.org/10.25259/SNI_241_2021.

27. Equitable access to state-of-the-art medical technology—a malaysian mini–public-private partnership case study. World Neurosurg 2022;157:135–42.

28. Haglund MM, Kiryabwire J, Parker S, et al. Surgical capacity building in Uganda through twinning, technology, and training camps. World J Surg 2011; 35(6). https://doi.org/10.1007/s00268-011-1080-0.

29. Waterkeyn F, Woodfield J, Massawe SL, et al. The effect of the Dar es Salaam neurosurgery training course on self-reported neurosurgical knowledge and confidence. Brain & spine 2023;3. https://doi.org/10.1016/j.bas.2023.101727.

30. Warf BC, Tracy S, Mugamba J. Long-term outcome for endoscopic third ventriculostomy alone or in combination with choroid plexus cauterization for congenital aqueductal stenosis in African infants. J Neurosurg Pediatr 2012;10(2):108–11.

31. Kulkarni AV, Schiff SJ, Mbabazi-Kabachelor E, et al. Endoscopic treatment versus shunting for infant hydrocephalus in Uganda. N Engl J Med 2017. https://doi.org/10.1056/NEJMoa1707568.

32. Haji FA, Lepard JR, Davis MC, et al. A model for global surgical training and capacity development: the Children's of Alabama-Viet Nam pediatric neurosurgery partnership. Childs Nerv Syst 2021;37(2): 627–36.

33. Rocque BG, Davis MC, McClugage SG, et al. Surgical treatment of epilepsy in Vietnam: program development and international collaboration. Neurosurg Focus 2018;45(4):E3.

34. Rock J, Glick R, Germano IM, et al. The first neurosurgery boot camp in southeast asia: evaluating impact on knowledge and regional collaboration in Yangon, Myanmar. World Neurosurg 2018;113: e239–46.

35. Tomycz LD, Markosian C, Kurilets I, et al. The co-pilot project: an international neurosurgical collaboration in Ukraine. World Neurosurg 2021;147. https://doi.org/10.1016/j.wneu.2020.12.100.

36. Dos Santos Rubio EJ, Calderon C, Boeykens A, et al. Can we build better? Challenges with geospatial and financial accessibility in the Caribbean. Illustrative case. Journal of neurosurgery Case lessons 2023;6(22). https://doi.org/10.3171/CASE23472.

37. Rolle ML, Williams A, Boeykens A, et al. Analysis of the Caribbean Neurosurgery Workforce: Scope of Practice, Challenges, and Ways Forward. World Neurosurg 2023;179. https://doi.org/10.1016/j.wneu.2023.08.039.

38. Paul AJ. Neurosurgery in Haiti: A Neglected Piece of the Healthcare Framework. BJSTR 2023;51(5): 43153–5.

39. Bowen I, Toor H, Zampella B, et al. Infrastructural limitations in establishing neurosurgical specialty services in Liberia. Cureus 2022;14(9). https://doi.org/10.7759/cureus.29373.

40. The Current State of Neurosurgery in Somaliland. World Neurosurg 2021;153:44–51.

41. Ammar A, Nawabi NLA, Hamzah R, et al. The current state of neurosurgery in Afghanistan. World Neurosurg 2023;169:110–7.e1.

42. Jumbam DT, Vervoort D, Park KB. Development Assistance for Health in Low-Income Countries. JAMA 2019;322(15):1517–8.

43. Kanmounye US, Robertson FC, Thango NS, et al. Needs of Young African Neurosurgeons and Residents: A Cross-Sectional Study. Front Surg 2021;8: 647279.

44. Barriers to Neurosurgical Training in Sub-Saharan Africa: The Need for a Phased Approach to Global Surgery Efforts to Improve Neurosurgical Care. World Neurosurg 2017;98:397–402.

45. Ferraris KP, Matsumura H, Wardhana DPW, et al. The state of neurosurgical training and education in East Asia: analysis and strategy development for this frontier of the world. Neurosurg Focus 2020;48(3):E7.

46. Murguia-Fuentes R, Husein N, Vega A, et al. Neurosurgical Residency Training in Latin America: Current Status, Challenges, and Future Opportunities. World Neurosurg 2018;120:e1079–97.

47. Karekezi C, El Khamlichi A, El Ouahabi A, et al. The impact of African-trained neurosurgeons on sub-Saharan Africa. Neurosurg Focus 2020;48(3):E4.

48. Tshimbombu TN, Kalubye AB, Hoffman C, et al. Review of Neurosurgery in the Democratic Republic of Congo: Historical Approach of a Local Context. World Neurosurg 2022;167. https://doi.org/10.1016/j.wneu.2022.07.113.

49. Beer-Furlan A, Neto SG, Teixeira MJ, et al. Fulfilling Need for Neurosurgical Services in Sub-Saharan Africa: Initial Angola-Brazil Training Experience. World Neurosurg 2019;122. https://doi.org/10.1016/j.wneu.2018.10.081.

50. Garba DL, Fadalla T, Sarpong K, et al. Access to training in neurosurgery (Part 2): The costs of pursuing neurosurgical training. Brain & Spine 2022;2. https://doi.org/10.1016/j.bas.2022.100927.

51. Westwick HJ, Elkaim LM, Obaid S, et al. Interest and participation in global neurosurgery: a survey of Canadian neurosurgery residents. Neurosurg Focus 2020;48(3):E21.

52. Nicolosi F, Rossini Z, Zaed I, et al. Neurosurgical digital teaching in low-middle income countries: beyond the frontiers of traditional education. Neurosurg Focus 2018;45(4):E17.

53. Takoutsing BD, Wunde UN, Zolo Y, et al. Assessing the impact of neurosurgery and neuroanatomy simulation using 3D non-cadaveric models amongst selected African medical students. Front Med Technol 2023;5: 1190096.

54. Ahmed R, Muirhead W, Williams SC, et al. A synthetic model simulator for intracranial aneurysm clipping: validation of the UpSurgeOn AneurysmBox. Front Surg 2023;10:1185516.

55. Hoffman C, Härtl R, Shlobin NA, et al. Future Directions for Global Clinical Neurosurgical Training: Challenges and Opportunities. World Neurosurg 2022; 166. https://doi.org/10.1016/j.wneu.2022.07.030.

56. Uche EO, Sundblom J, Iloabachie I, et al. Pilot application of Lecture-Panel-Discussion Model (LPDM) in global collaborative neurosurgical education: a novel training paradigm innovated by the Swedish African Neurosurgery Collaboration. Acta Neurochir 2022;164(4):967.

57. Gerstl JVE, Blitz SE, Qu QR, et al. Global, Regional, and National Economic Consequences of Stroke. Stroke 2023;54(9). https://doi.org/10.1161/STROKEAHA.123.043131.

58. Lartigue JW, Dada OE, Haq M, et al. Emphasizing the Role of Neurosurgery Within Global Health and National Health Systems: A Call to Action. Front Surg 2021;8:690735.

59. Garcia RM, Ghotme KA, Arynchyna-Smith A, et al. Global Neurosurgery: Progress and Resolutions at the 75th World Health Assembly. Neurosurgery 2023. https://doi.org/10.1227/neu.0000000000002472.

60. Gupta S, Aukrust CG, Bhebhe A, et al. Neurosurgery and the World Health Organization Intersectoral Global Action Plan for Epilepsy and Other Neurological Disorders 2022-2031. Neurosurgery 2024. https://doi.org/10.1227/neu.0000000000002828.

Postgraduate Fellowships, Distant Continuing Education, and Funding in Neurosurgical Education

Ignatius N. Esene, MD, PhD, MPH[a,b,c], Juliet Sekabunga, MD[a,d],
Robert J. Dempsey, MD[a,e],*

KEYWORDS

• Distant continuing education • Funding • Postgraduate fellowships • Neurosurgery

KEY POINTS

• Education and training are the essential tenets for sustainable neurosurgical care system.
• Opportunities for neurosurgical training are limited due to socioeconomic constraints and an inadequate workforce.
• There has been a recent huge drive to expand training opportunities to cater for this unmet need.
• Most training programs especially those in developing settings are focused on basic residency training with no opportunities for fellowships and continuing education.
• The Foundation of International Education in Neurological Surgery is a global success model to elucidate on the role of fellowships, distant continuing education, and funding in neurosurgical education.

INTRODUCTION

Neurosurgical education and training are the essential tenets for the development of a sustainable workforce: the core of an optimal neurosurgical care system. However, opportunities for neurosurgical training are limited in most parts of the world due to socioeconomic constraints and an inadequate workforce. This global deficit of about 23,500 neurosurgeons to provide at least 5 million essential neurosurgery procedures in the last decades has led to the huge drive to expand training opportunities to cater for this unmet need. The number of training programs has witnessed a steady increase especially in high-income countries. However, most of these programs especially those in developing settings are focused on basic residency training with no opportunities for fellowships and continuing education. Trainees in these resource-limited settings have to travel during or after their residency for fellowships in high-income countries for additional training. Those who cannot afford the luxury of traveling are reliant on distant continuing education. In this succinct review, we use the Foundation of International Education in Neurological Surgery (FIENS) as a global success model to elucidate on the role of fellowships, distant continuing education, and funding in neurosurgical education.

---

[a] Foundation for International Education in Neurological Surgery (FIENS); [b] Faculty of Health Sciences, University of Bamenda, Bambili, Cameroon; [c] Winners Foundation, Yaounde, Cameroon; [d] Mulago National Referral Hospital, Kampala, Uganda; [e] Department of Neurological Surgery, University of Wisconsin School of Medicine and Public Health, Madison, WI, USA
* Corresponding author. Department of Neurological Surgery, University of Wisconsin School of Medicine and Public Health, Madison, WI.
E-mail address: dempsey@neurosurgery.wisc.edu

Neurosurg Clin N Am 35 (2024) 499–507
https://doi.org/10.1016/j.nec.2024.05.012
1042-3680/24/© 2024 Elsevier Inc. All rights are reserved, including those for text and data mining, AI training, and similar technologies.

CONTINUING EDUCATION IN MEDICINE AND NEUROSURGERY

Continuing education encompasses a wide range of knowledge and skills acquisition for professionals in various fields following completion of formal training.[1] It has several appellations including "lifelong learning," "continuing medical education," "professional education," "career enrichment," and "skill development."[2] It entails programs, courses, and activities aimed at taking curriculum-based university degree programs to the next levels, making them more accessible and allowing professionals to stay abreast with current standards and trends in their respective fields. It plays a crucial role in helping professionals enhance their skills, maintain compliance, and adapt to the evolving demands of their professional milieu.[3] Continuing education follows the precept that professionals are continuous learners looking to expand on their already enriched knowledge.[1] As a result, these courses are not basic, but rather supplementary. They are offered by universities, professional organizations, and through many other educational sources depending on the field and can be disseminated virtually or onsite. These providers collaborate with experts in different fields to develop and deliver educational content. Despite being supplementary in nature, fields such as teaching and health care often have continuing education compulsory as a requirement to enroll in certain programs or imposed by licensing bodies for certain employment positions.[4] Continuing education can be delivered in the form of conferences, seminars/webinars, journal clubs, courses, grand rounds, on-the-job training, traditional classroom settings, or self-assessment modules.[5] With the advent of the COVID-19 pandemic and in war-torn parts of the world, there has been a marked shift in the utilization of information and communication technologies to facilitate learning in various study modalities and teaching–learning processes.

Continuing education in health care also called continuing medical education (CME) has its own standard and application. It is aimed at improving the quality of health care and maintaining the doctors and paramedical team ability to provide quality patient care.[6] It also ensures they stay updated with the latest advancements, research, and best practices in the field of medicine. Given its importance, and the need to guarantee the quality, relevance, and scientific rigor of the educational content, it is important to have independent professional bodies responsible for assessing and ensuring consistent quality across all CME activities.[7] Often CME is given by approved educational offerings. National organizations charged with the approval of CME enforce that by making it a requirement for renewal of medical license-ship (licensing certification to practice) or specialized board certification for subspecialties. In the United States, for example, the American Medical Association and the Accreditation Council for Continuing Medical Education have played a significant role in the development of guidelines for good medical practice and the establishment of mandatory continuing education programs. CME programs and providers are often accredited to ensure they meet certain quality standards.[8] They provide opportunities to learn from experts and engage in provoking discussions. They cover a wide range of medical topics and are often tailored to different specialties, with some being specific and others broad.[9] The topics are often tailored to different specialties and areas of interest. In addition, some medical specialties have specific maintenance requiring health care actors to complete a combination of continuing education activities, self-assessment modules, and performance assessments to demonstrate ongoing competence.[10] This may vary between countries, and health care professionals working in international settings may need to comply with the specific requirements of the country they are practicing in or the organization they are affiliated with.

Continuing education goes beyond clinical knowledge and skills. It also addresses broader professional development areas, such as communication skills, leadership, cultural competence, and ethics.[11] These topics are crucial for health care professionals to provide patient-centered care, collaborate effectively with colleagues, and navigate complex ethical dilemmas such as that frequently encountered in neurosurgery practice.[12] Attending CME programs requires dedication and can be challenging for busy health care professionals.[13] Additionally, some programs exhibit significant cost; however, many programs offer full or partial waiver for students, those with disabilities as well as those originating from low- and middle-income countries (LMICs). Access to high-quality continuing education may be limited, particularly for health care professionals practicing in rural or remote areas. However, there has been a fast adoption of virtual platforms heightened by the recent pandemics to overcome this. Traditional programs often follow a didactic format, with presentations and lectures dominating the learning experience.[14] This passive learning approach may not fully engage participants or promote active knowledge acquisition and critical thinking. Alternative learning methods, such as case-based discussions, interactive workshops, and simulation-based training, have proved to be more effective in enhancing health care providers' engagement and ease application in real-world settings when caring for patients. Some programs use a credit system to quantify the educational value of each activity with one credit typically representing 1 hour of educational content.[15] The number of credits required for licensure or certification renewal varies by jurisdiction and specialty. Some activities receive funding or support from companies and stakeholders, raising concerns about potential bias or conflicts of interest.[16] Given the strict adherence to ethical principles, it is important for health care professionals to critically evaluate the content to ensure they receive balanced and evidence-based education.

Neurosurgeons, like all physicians, are required to participate in CME to stay up-to-date on the latest advancements and best practices in their field.[17] CME could be accorded more importance than licensing regulation because it affects the quality of the ongoing education in each person's personal professional development. The field of neurosurgery having its own unique challenges, techniques, and subspecialties; therefore, CME activities in neurosurgery are tailored to address these specific needs.[18] They cover a wide range of topics, including neurosciences, neuroradiology, neuro-oncology, neurotrauma, neurocritical care, neurovascular surgery, spine surgery, pediatric neurosurgery, functional neurosurgery, and more. Professional neurosurgical organizations and societies, such as the American Association of Neurological Surgeons, the Congress of Neurological Surgeons, the European Association of Neurosurgical Societies, and the World Federation of Neurosurgical Societies organize annual meetings and conferences.[19] They often qualify for CME credits and serve as a medium for neurosurgeons to engage in scientific discussions, attend educational sessions, participate in hands-on workshops, and present their research. Given the technical expertise and precision required in neurosurgery, hands-on workshops and simulation training provide opportunities for neurosurgeons to practice and refine their surgical skills in a controlled environment. These workshops cover various neurosurgical techniques, including endoscopic, micro, and minimal invasive neurosurgery. Virtual platforms dedicated to neurosurgery provide access to a wide range of educational resources.[20] These media are usually flexible, allowing neurosurgeons to learn at their own pace dependless of their location. In addition, neurosurgery subspecialty CME activities allow neurosurgeons to delve deeper into their areas of interest and gain specialized knowledge and skills.

Many neurosurgeons are required to participate in a "Maintenance of Certification" program to maintain their board certification. This involves a combination of CME activities, self-assessment modules, and performance assessments to demonstrate ongoing competence in neurosurgery.[21]

In low-resource settings, neurosurgery CME can be challenging due to limited access to training programs and financial constraints. CME in this setting are usually in the form of training during workshops and conferences or through online courses and usually do not offer CME credits.[22] Given the high cost of such training with the standard on high-income countries, many accessible media and resources have been used to address this issue. One approach is the use of low-cost exoscopic visualization systems for surgical training, which have been shown to be safe and feasible for procedures such as lumbar interbody fusions in low-resource settings.[23] Another option is the incorporation of free, web-based, 3 dimensional visualization apps for patient education, which can provide better understanding of complex neurosurgical diseases and procedures. Neurosimulation training using noncadaveric models has also proven a significant impact in improving practical neuroanatomy and neurosurgery knowledge.[24] Also, microscopic and endoscopic training for complex brain and spine surgeries has proven to be effective. Additionally, virtual reality interfaces have been utilized to provide real-time guidance and training for emergency neurosurgical procedures, enabling remote proctorship and access to expertise.[25] These innovative approaches have the potential to improve access to neurosurgical training and education in low-resource settings, bridging the gap and enhancing patient care.

The FIENS (https://fiens.org/) is actively involved in providing neurosurgical CME opportunities. It offers hands-on training, education, and volunteer programs to neurosurgeons globally, focusing on addressing the critical shortage of trained neurosurgeons in LMICs.[26] Through initiatives such as boot camps and virtual training programs, FIENS aims to enhance neurosurgical education and training on an international scale. This commitment to education and training underscores FIENS' dedication to improving health care outcomes and building neurosurgical capacity worldwide. FIENS CME programs are tailored to neurosurgeons and trainees worldwide. It aims to provide ongoing learning, skill development, and knowledge enhancement in the field of neurosurgery.[26] FIENS may offer online courses and webinars in the form of "Virtual Visiting Professor Webinar" covering various topics in neurosurgery, including surgical techniques for neurosurgical pathologies, history, and leadership in neurosurgery among others. The interactivity of the sessions allows participants, especially fellows to learn from experts in the field and engage into provocative discussions. Its platform offers curated content, case studies, video lectures, and other educational materials accessible anytime, and anywhere. Also, international boot camps in South America, Asia, and Africa have served as an important source of CME. Educational materials include mini courses with lectures, case discussions, skill stations, simulators, and models. This form of CME also provides an opportunity for global north–south networking and learning about up-to-date techniques and equipment in neurosurgery. FIENS works in collaboration with other organizations, institutions, and academic institutions in the development and delivery of CME materials. These collaborative partnerships usually come as a result of joint conferences, educational initiatives, or research projects with a neurosurgical theme (**Fig. 1**). Also, some of its CME activities are accredited or certified by recognized accrediting bodies or professional organizations, ensuring that participants receive credit or certification for their participation in CME sessions.

FELLOWSHIPS IN NEUROSURGERY

Access to opportunities for professional development and advanced education is more important than ever. Professional development and advanced education are crucial today as global changes happen fast. On this path of growth, financial issues and geographic barriers are a major source of hindrance. However, hope shines through difficulties as fellowships offer a path to the continuous learning journey, opening doors for aspirations to becoming a reality.[27] Fellowships are prestigious awards that go to health professionals or scholars to support advanced training.[28] They support research professional development focusing on a specific field or discipline. These opportunities are highly competitive, and recipients get chosen on merit with academic excellence and impact to the society being a major selection criteria.[29]

Fellowships provide a financial support which includes tuition fee waivers, living expenses, travel cost, and research materials among others. In addition, fellows gain other benefits such as increased access to specialized facilities, mentorship from field experts, and networking. One primary purpose of fellowships is for expertise deepening, enabling acquisition of new skills and undertaking innovative research projects. All of which contribute to knowledge advancement in respective medical specialties. Fellowships offer a structured environment for focused, independent training or research to improve clinical practice, health outcomes, and quality of life and this happens under the guidance of experienced mentors. Fellowships foster collaboration and idea exchange among diverse scholars or professionals. This leads to interdisciplinary approaches and breakthrough discoveries. Fellowships nurture talent, promote excellence, and drive innovation across various fields, ultimately contributing indirectly to societal progress and development. For residents of LMICs, fellowships are transformative opportunities.[30] They provide access to advanced training in cutting-edge techniques not available locally and facilitate research at the frontiers of knowledge. They elevate the skills and subject mastery of recipients with far-reaching positive impacts felt beyond the fellow. This includes strengthening the health care workforce and systems and improved patient care, health outcomes in underserved regions of the world.

In the surgical realm, fellowships shape the future of specialities such as neurosurgery.[31] Neurosurgery fellows undergo rigorous specialized training in complex procedures. Hands-on experience operating under expert guidance is a core component. They gain exposure to the latest innovative surgical techniques and technologies. Through close mentorship by esteemed neurosurgeons, fellows refine their skills and master intricate brain and spinal surgeries.[32] Extensive collaboration with leading neurosurgeons facilitates expertise development for fellows. By pushing boundaries, they advance neurosurgical capabilities, standards of

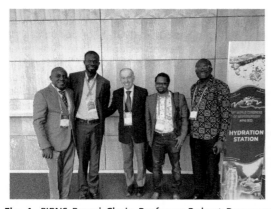

Fig. 1. FIENS Board Chair, Professor Robert Dempsey (*Middle*) with some FIENS alumni. (From *left*) Dr Ignatius Esene (Cameroon) and Dr Yannick Canton (Chad) and young FIENS members. (From *right*) Dr Alvin Doe (Liberia) and Dr Luxwell Jokonya (Zimbabwe) at the World Neurosurgery Congress in Cape Town.

practice, and ultimately enhance patient care and treatment outcomes. The ripple effects of neurosurgery fellowships extend far beyond the individual journeys of their recipients.[33] Across continents, these programs propel advancements in surgical techniques, pushing the boundaries of what was once thought impossible. They fuel groundbreaking research endeavors, shaping the very landscape of this intricate field. Fellowships also enrich educational initiatives worldwide, ensuring the dissemination of cutting-edge knowledge to the next generation. In the dynamic realm of neurosurgery, where precision and technical mastery are paramount, fellowships cultivate excellence like few other avenues can. They nurture the development of highly skilled surgeons, instilling in them a relentless pursuit of expertise. The influence of these programs transcends borders, propelling overall progress within this critically important specialty. Neurosurgery fellowships resonate globally, with their impact far exceeding individual trajectories.[34] These prestigious opportunities catalyze innovations in surgical approaches and technologies, ushering in new eras of treatment possibilities. They provide fertile ground for pioneering research that expands the very boundaries of what we understand about the human brain and nervous system. Simultaneously, fellowships elevate educational standards and curricula internationally, ensuring a continuous cycle of knowledge transfer.[35] These programs shape the future leaders of neurosurgery–the eminent academicians and clinicians who will guide the field forward. They instill a mindset of continuous learning and improvement, driving transformative advances that redefine neurosurgical practice time and again.

An example of neurosurgery fellowship with significant impact is the FIENS (https://fiens.org/) Fellow Program.

FIENS offer fellowships to neurosurgeons and trainees in LMICs without sufficient neurosurgical coverage to enhance their skills and knowledge in the field of neurosurgery. These fellowships provide a valuable opportunity for neurosurgeons to observe and learn from experienced professionals, facilitating the rapid transfer of knowledge and expertise.[36] FIENS offers visiting fellowships (Bassett and Clack Global Neurosurgery Fellowships) for neurosurgeons who come from or are training in LMICs. Its fellowship programs focus on the creation of sustainable training programs in partnership with host organizations, emphasizing on local neurosurgery resident education and the development of neurosurgery residency program. This is in recognition of the need for ongoing support for trainees in the early stages of their careers. Through these initiatives, FIENS

aims to amplify the overall impact of its efforts and contribute to the development of self-sustaining health systems in regions of need. The fellowship program offered by the FIENS exists in the form of clinical, research, global health, ethics and humanitarian, subspecialty, and educational fellowships. The research fellowship program aims at advancing scientific knowledge and innovation in neurosurgery with a focus on low-resource settings (global neurosurgery).

Research fellows have the opportunity to conduct research projects under the guidance of leading neurosurgical researchers, contributing to advancements in understanding neurosurgical diseases, treatment outcomes, and surgical techniques. Clinical fellowship on the other hand focuses on providing hands-on clinical experience in specific areas of neurosurgery. This includes general and pediatric neurosurgery, neurotrauma, skull base, cerebrovascular neurosurgery, and neuro-oncology.

Clinical fellows are either trainees or recently trained neurosurgeons working closely with experienced consultants, gaining practical skills and expertise in their chosen subspecialty areas of interest. Educational fellowships focus on training neurosurgical educators and leaders who are dedicated to advancing neurosurgical education and training programs in their home countries or regions. These fellowships involve mentorship, curriculum development, teaching workshops, or educational research projects aimed at enhancing the quality of neurosurgical education globally (**Fig. 2**A–C).

Funding Continuing Education and Fellowships in Neurosurgery

Funding education and medical training is an indispensable investment for the overall well-being and progress of our current society.[37] By ensuring that students and trainees receive quality education by supporting them with adequate resources, we cultivate a skilled and knowledgeable workforce. This will ensure that there are enough seasoned health care professionals to meet the needs of the population, thus contributing to better health care outcomes and an improved quality of life for patients.[38] Funding primarily enables educational institutions to improve education access for a broader range of students. This funding can be dispensed on formal training, or through CME, and fellowships. Funding for CME and fellowships in particular is crucial for the professional development of health care providers and the advancement of medical knowledge.[3] It contributes to improving educational and health care infrastructure,

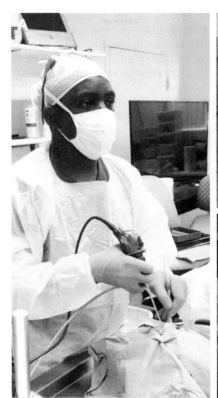
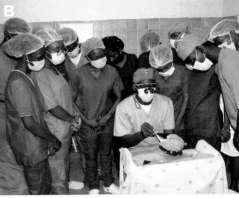
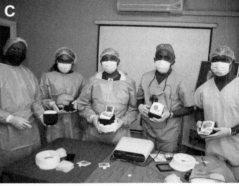

Fig. 2. FIENS Basset fellow alumni (Dr Ignatius Esene) learning endoscopic skills in Wisconsin (*A*). Training of medical students (*B*) and young neurosurgeons in neurosimulation (*C*) in Cameroon.

curriculum development, research facilities, and the integration of technology. These funding opportunities facilitate access to specialized training, workshops, conferences, and educational resources which may not be readily available through traditional means especially for professionals practicing in LMICs. Moreover, funding CME and fellowships in the domain of neurosurgery contributes to the overall quality of health care delivery by promoting evidence-based neurosurgical practices, ethical standards, patient safety protocols, and ultimately improving neurosurgical health outcomes.[39]

Funding neurosurgery research fellowship in particular contributes to the execution of groundbreaking research that leads to surgical breakthroughs, new treatments, and advancements in health care technology for neurosurgery.[40] Furthermore, the financial support for fellowships and CME is instrumental in cultivating future leaders in neurosurgical training. By investing in faculty development and educational leadership programs, institutions can ensure a continuous cycle of improvement in the quality of neurosurgical education, curriculum design, assessment methods, and neurosurgery program evaluation.[41] Investing in educational leadership ultimately

benefits aspiring neurosurgeons, neurosurgery residents, and consultants by fostering a culture of excellence and innovation in medical training.[42] It can also stimulate economic growth. This is because a skilled workforce attracts top businesses and industries that rely on highly trained professionals. Additionally, it can lead to the creation of new industries and job opportunities, further contributing to economic development. Countries investing in CME and fellowships (leadership, research, or clinical) are prone to being competitive on a global scale.[10] A well-educated workforce and a robust health care system enhance a country's competitiveness by improving productivity, innovation, public health preparedness in times of crises such as pandemics or natural disasters, and overall quality of life.[43] Last, funding neurosurgery fellowships can help address gaps and inequities in health care by training professionals in neurosurgical subspecialties that are in high demand but have scarce workforce specially in LMICs.[44] In LMICs, this will help attract specialization in the field and reduce the brain drain of health care providers in these communities, improving access to care for underserved populations.

The sources of funding for CME and fellowships in neurosurgery vary, some from out-of-pocket paying or receiving funding from their institutions.[45] Other funding sources include neurosurgery-oriented associations and societies, government and industry support, philanthropic donations, and nonprofit organizations and foundations.[45] Despite this, availability of sponsorship and eligibility criteria can vary widely depending on factors such as geographic location, medical specialty, career stage, and potential for impact and leadership.[36] Thus, the process can be competitive and offered to best applicants decided by a selection committee or board members. It is therefore important for neurologic surgeons, residents, and neurosurgery aspirants interested in pursuing funding for CME and fellowships to search specific opportunities and explore the resources available through their institutions, professional networks, and relevant funding bodies.

FIENS provides funding via scholarships for various initiatives aimed at advancing neurosurgical education, training, research, and patient care worldwide especially in LMICs. It offers financial support for neurosurgeons to pursue specialized training through fellowships in various subspecialties of neurosurgery (Bassett Global Neurosurgery Fellowship). This funding may cover stipends, travel expenses, accommodation, and other costs associated with the fellowship program.[46] It also provides funding in the form of scholarships, to support neurosurgical trainees in developing countries to finish their neurosurgical training so that they may provide care in their home country (Clack Family Scholarship) (www. fiens.org). FIENS makes funding available with the help of collaborators and donations to support CME activities in LMICs. FIENS provides funding through grants for research projects aimed at advancing scientific understanding and innovation in neurosurgery. These grants support investigations into neurosurgical diseases, treatment outcomes, surgical techniques, and other areas of interest to the neurosurgical community.

SUMMARY

Neurosurgical education and training stands at the forefront of ensuring optimal neurosurgical care globally. Despite significant progress, challenges persist, particularly in resource-limited settings where opportunities for training are scarce. CME in neurosurgery plays a crucial role in keeping neurosurgeons updated with the latest advancements and best practices in their field. Moreover, by providing opportunities for advanced training, research, and collaboration, fellowships contribute to the development of highly skilled neurosurgeons who can address complex surgical challenges and improve patient outcomes. Investing in education and training in neurosurgery is not only an investment in the health care workforce but also enhancing health care delivery, fostering innovation, and promoting economic growth and societal development. Funding support for CME and fellowships is crucial for advancing medical knowledge, promoting innovation, and addressing health care disparities worldwide. By ensuring access to quality education and training opportunities, we can cultivate a skilled workforce, drive advancements in neurosurgical care, and ultimately improve health outcomes for patients globally. FIENS stands out as a global success model, serving as a cornerstone for lifelong learning, skill enhancement, and funding among neurosurgeons and trainees, especially in LMICs. Through its initiatives, it facilitates access to high-quality education regardless of geographic constraints. By collaborating with other organizations and accrediting bodies, FIENS ensures the delivery of evidence-based and ethically sound educational content. These prestigious awards provide financial support, specialized training, mentorship, and networking opportunities, ultimately shaping the future leaders and innovators in the field of neurosurgery.

DISCLOSURE

The authors have nothing to disclose.

REFERENCES

1. Gallagher L. Continuing education in nursing: A concept analysis. Nurse Educ Today 2007;27(5): 466–73.
2. Laal M, Laal A, Aliramaei A. Continuing Education; Lifelong Learning. Procedia - Social and Behavioral Sciences 2014;116:4052–6.
3. Sysoieva S, Protsenko O. Implementation of the continuing education concept in the european educational area: regulatory provision. Continuing Professional Education: Theory and Practice 2020; 0(2):78–84.
4. Mlambo M, Silen C, McGrath C. Lifelong learning and nurses' continuing professional development, a metasynthesis of the literature. BMC Nurs 2021; 20(1):62.
5. Forsetlund L, O'Brien MA, Forsen L, et al. Continuing education meetings and workshops: effects on professional practice and healthcare outcomes. Cochrane Database Syst Rev 2021;9(9):CD003030.

6. Kluwer W., What is continuing medical education and why do I need it? 2018. Available at: https://www.wolterskluwer.com/en/expert-insights/what-is-continuing-medical-education-and-why-do-i-need-it.

7. Blodgett A. CME activity guidelines: university at buffalo. Jacobs School of Medicine and Biomedical, 2024 Biomedical Sciences; 2024. Available at: https://medicine.buffalo.edu/cme/planning_cme/plan_non_recurring/cme_activity_guidelines.html.

8. Zarei M, Mojarrab S, Bazrafkan L, et al. The role of continuing medical education programs in promoting iranian nurses, competency toward non-communicable diseases, a qualitative content analysis study. BMC Med Educ 2022;22(1):731.

9. Price DW, Davis DA, Filerman GL. "Systems-Integrated CME": The Implementation and Outcomes Imperative for Continuing Medical Education in the Learning Health Care Enterprise. NAM Perspect 2021;2021.

10. Alameri HF, McMahon GT, Al Jenaibi FH, et al. Abu Dhabi's Journey Towards Excellence in Continuing Medical Education. Journal of CME 2023;12(1):2285381.

11. Samuel A, Cervero RM, Durning SJ, et al. Effect of Continuing Professional Development on Health Professionals' Performance and Patient Outcomes: A Scoping Review of Knowledge Syntheses. Acad Med 2021;96(6):913–23.

12. Shlobin NA, Sheldon M, Lam S. Informed consent in neurosurgery: a systematic review. Neurosurg Focus 2020;49(5):E6.

13. Setia S, Tay JC, Chia YC, et al. Massive open online courses (MOOCs) for continuing medical education – why and how? Adv Med Educ Pract 2019;10(null):805–12.

14. Sivarajah RT, Curci NE, Johnson EM, et al. A Review of Innovative Teaching Methods. Acad Radiol 2019;26(1):101–13.

15. Pardos ZA, Borchers C, Yu R. Credit hours is not enough: Explaining undergraduate perceptions of course workload using LMS records. Internet High Educ 2023;56:100882.

16. Barnes B. Financial conflicts of interest in continuing medical education: implications and accountability. JAMA 2017;317(17):1741–2.

17. Ammar A, Bernstein M. Neurosurgeons' duties. In: Ammar A, Bernstein M, editors. Neurosurgical ethics in practice: value-based medicine. Berlin, Heidelberg: Springer Berlin Heidelberg; 2014. p. 123–34.

18. Hoffman C, Hartl R, Shlobin NA, et al. Future directions for global clinical neurosurgical training: challenges and opportunities. World Neurosurgery 2022;166:e404–18.

19. Araujo AVS, Lacerda AA, Oliveira AA, et al. Neurosurgery societies around the world: A study and discussion about its importance. Surg Neurol Int 2023;14:161.

20. Stienen MN, Schaller K, Cock H, et al. eLearning resources to supplement postgraduate neurosurgery training. Acta Neurochir 2017;159(2):325–37.

21. Babu MA, Liau LM, Connolly ES, et al. Maintenance of certification: perceptions and attitudes of neurosurgeons. Neurosurgery 2018;83(4):835–42.

22. Maria NU. Enhancing neurosurgical education in low- and middle-income countries with financial constraints through web-based learning. J Neurol Surg B Skull Base 2022;83(S 01):P150.

23. Ramirez ME, Peralta I, Nurmukhametov R, et al. Expanding access to microneurosurgery in low-resource settings: Feasibility of a low-cost exoscope in transforaminal lumbar interbody fusion. J Neurosci Rural Pract 2023;14(1):156–60.

24. Takoutsing BD, Wunde UN, Zolo Y, et al. Assessing the impact of neurosurgery and neuroanatomy simulation using 3D non-cadaveric models amongst selected African medical students. Front Med Technol 2023;5:1190096.

25. Please H, Edemaga D, Bolton W, et al. 4 Using virtual reality to deliver essential neurosurgery in austere and low-resource settings. BMJ Military Health 2023;169(2):e1.

26. Mosberg WH, Svien HJ, Tyrer AR, et al. Foundation for international education in neurological surgery, incorporated. J Neurosurg 1970;33(5):481–4.

27. Rajan S, Luoma AMV, Kofke WA. Role of fellowship training in furthering innovations in perioperative neuroscience. J Neurosurg Anesthesiol 2024;36(1):1–3.

28. Stern S. Fellowship training: a necessity in today's academic world. Acad Emerg Med 2002;9(7):713–6.

29. Grover BT, Kothari SN. Fellowship Training: Need and Contributions. Surg Clin North Am 2016;96(1):47–57.

30. Käser M, Maure C, Halpaap BM, et al. Research Capacity Strengthening in Low and Middle Income Countries - An Evaluation of the WHO/TDR Career Development Fellowship Programme. PLoS Negl Trop Dis 2016;10(5):e0004631.

31. Sarpong K, Fadalla T, Garba DL, et al. Access to training in neurosurgery (Part 1): Global perspectives and contributing factors of barriers to access. Brain Spine 2022;2:100900.

32. Kaba M, Birhanu Z, Fernandez Villalobos NV, et al. Health research mentorship in low- and middle-income countries: a scoping review. JBI Evid Synth 2023;21(10):1912–70.

33. Wang K, Bhandarkar AR, Bauman MMJ, et al. International trends in grant and fellowship funding awarded to women in neurosurgery. Neurosurg Focus 2021;50(3):E5.

34. Dupepe EB, Kicielinski KP, Gordon AS, et al. What is a case-control study? Neurosurgery 2019;84(4):819–26.

35. Selden NR, Barbaro NM, Barrow DL, et al. Neurosurgery residency and fellowship education in the

United States: 2 decades of system development by the One Neurosurgery Summit organizations. J Neurosurg 2022;136(2):565–74.

36. Dempsey RJ. Editorial. Global neurosurgery: the role of the individual neurosurgeon, the Foundation for International Education in Neurological Surgery, and "service through education" to address worldwide need. Neurosurg Focus 2018;45(4):E19.

37. Stephane V, Pratibha G, Iman A, et al. Investing in school systems: conceptualising returns on investment across the health, education and social protection sectors. BMJ Glob Health 2023;8(12):e012545.

38. Worsley C, Webb S, Vaux E. Training healthcare professionals in quality improvement. Future Hosp J 2016;3(3):207–10.

39. Spithoff S. Industry involvement in continuing medical education: time to say no. Can Fam Physician 2014;60(8):700–3.

40. ReFaey K, Freeman WD, Tripathi S, et al. NIH funding trends for neurosurgeon-scientists from 1993-2017: Biomedical workforce implications for neuro-oncology. J Neuro Oncol 2021;154(1):51–62.

41. Yong RL, Cheung W, Shrivastava RK, et al. Teaching quality in neurosurgery: quantitating outcomes over time. J Neurosurg 2022;136(4):1147–56.

42. Neal MT, Lyons MK. Empowering qualities and skills for leaders in neurosurgery. Surg Neurol Int 2021;12:9.

43. Dempsey KE, Qureshi MM, Ondoma SM, et al. Effect of Geopolitical Forces on Neurosurgical Training in Sub-Saharan Africa. World Neurosurg 2017;101:196–202.

44. Barthelemy EJ, Diouf SA, Silva ACV, et al. Historical determinants of neurosurgical inequities in Africa and the African diaspora: A review and analysis of coloniality. PLOS Glob Public Health 2023;3(2):e0001550.

45. Venkataraman R, Ranganathan L, Ponnish AS, et al. Funding sources for continuing medical education: An observational study. Indian J Crit Care Med 2014;18(8):513–7.

46. Mosberg WH. Foundation for international education in neurological surgery, incorporated. J Neurosurg 1970;33(5):481–4.

Training the Next Generation of Academic Neurosurgeons in Global Health, Academics, and Research

Anthony T. Fuller, MD, MScGH[a,b,1],
Michael M. Haglund, MD, PhD, MEd, MACM[a,c,d],*

KEYWORDS

- Global neurosurgery • Health equity • Interdisciplinary collaboration • Research innovation
- Training and education • Sustainable partnerships

KEY POINTS

- Academic global neurosurgeons blend surgical expertise with global health principles to address disparities in neurosurgical care worldwide.
- Comprehensive training that includes global health, research, and leadership skills is essential for cultivating the next generation of academic global neurosurgeons.
- Interdisciplinary collaboration and cultural humility are crucial for implementing effective and sustainable health interventions in diverse settings.
- Establishing long-term, equitable partnerships with local communities and health care systems is foundational to the success of global neurosurgery initiatives.

INTRODUCTION

Since its inception as a field, neurosurgery has inherently been a specialty where clinical expertise intermingled with academic pursuits. Thus, many neurosurgeons today consider themselves academic neurosurgeons, where their day-to-day shifts from the clinic to the operating room as quickly as it does from laboratory research to conference presentation. Within the past few decades, a global orientation within neurosurgery has emerged, with the field of global neurosurgery taking off exponentially within the past 10 to 15 years.[1–3] Global neurosurgery is commonly defined, although admittedly broadly,[4] as "an area for study, research, practice, and advocacy that places priority on improving health outcomes and achieving health equity for all people worldwide who are affected by neurosurgical conditions or have a need for neurosurgical care."[5] With this definition in mind, there is a need to consider how the next generation of neurosurgeons will be trained to become academic global neurosurgeons, what their training should entail, how to integrate it within current training, and how to reimagine academic positions posttraining.

Academic Global Neurosurgeons

An academic global neurosurgeon represents a transformative figure in the medical world, combining

a Duke Global Neurosurgery and Neurology, Durham, NC, USA; b Fuller Health Solutions, Salt Lake City, UT, USA; c Duke University Global Health Institute, Durham, NC, USA; d Department of Neurosurgery, Duke Health, Durham, NC, USA
1 Present address: 250 East 200 South, 15-112, Salt Lake City, UT 84111.
* Corresponding author. 4508 Hospital South, Durham, NC 27710.
E-mail address: michael.haglund@duke.edu

Neurosurg Clin N Am 35 (2024) 509–518
https://doi.org/10.1016/j.nec.2024.05.013
1042-3680/24/© 2024 Elsevier Inc. All rights reserved, including those for text and data mining, AI training, and similar technologies.

the precision of neurosurgery with the broad-reaching visions of global health initiatives. These professionals are distinguished by their surgical expertise and unwavering commitment to addressing the complex health challenges that transcend national borders and socioeconomic divides. Their study is rooted in the belief that medical knowledge and skills should serve as universal assets, freely crossing geographic and cultural barriers to alleviate suffering and promote health equity. By integrating research and education into their clinical practice, they push the boundaries of what is possible in medicine, advocating for innovative solutions to neurologic health disparities and fostering environments where knowledge and resources are shared for the common good.

The role of an academic global neurosurgeon extends far beyond the traditional scope of surgical care, encompassing a broad spectrum of responsibilities that include mentorship, policy advocacy, and cross-cultural collaboration.[6] They are at the forefront of developing and implementing training programs to empower local health care professionals in underserved regions, thereby building sustainable health care infrastructures.[7-11] Through collaborative research projects, they investigate the epidemiology of neurologic disorders across different populations, aiming to understand and mitigate the factors contributing to disparities in neurosurgical care.[12-14] Their leadership in global health initiatives often leads them to engage with policymakers and international health organizations, advocating for changes prioritizing the needs of the most vulnerable populations.[15-17]

Furthermore, academic global neurosurgeons embody a spirit of innovation and resilience, navigating the challenges of delivering high-quality neurosurgical care in resource-limited settings. They are pioneers in adapting and inventing surgical techniques and technologies that are both effective and accessible, ensuring that advancements in neurosurgery reach those in dire need.[18] Their study is a testament to the power of combining medical expertise with a deep commitment to global health equity, inspiring future generations of health care professionals. Therefore, the academic global neurosurgeon is not only a surgical practitioner but also a global health diplomat, striving to forge a future where every individual, regardless of where they are born, has access to the life-saving care they deserve.

care access and provider availability.[19-22] These disparities are not mere statistics but represent countless individuals deprived of the chance for treatment, recovery, and a life free from the burden of neurologic disorders. In regions where health care systems are overwhelmed or underresourced, the expertise and leadership of academic global neurosurgeons can catalyze significant improvements. By integrating their clinical practice with a deep understanding of public health principles, they are uniquely positioned to address not only the immediate needs of patients but also the systemic issues that perpetuate inequity. Their study in training, research, and policy advocacy is critical in elevating the standards of care and making neurosurgical interventions more accessible and effective for all, irrespective of geography or socioeconomic status.

Furthermore, academic global neurosurgeons play a pivotal role in the global health ecosystem by fostering international collaborations and knowledge exchange.[23-25] They are vital links among disparate health care systems, enabling the flow of innovations, best practices, and resources across borders. This collaborative approach is essential in tackling global health challenges that are too complex for any single entity to address alone. Through partnerships with local health care providers, governments, and international organizations, academic global neurosurgeons help to build capacity and resilience within health care systems. Their commitment to mentorship and education ensures that the next generation of health care professionals is equipped with the skills and knowledge to continue advancing the cause of health equity.[26-29]

Moreover, academic global neurosurgeons embody the principle that health care innovation should benefit everyone, not just those in affluent or developed regions. They are instrumental in driving research that prioritizes the development of cost-effective, scalable solutions to neurosurgical challenges faced by low and middle-income countries (LMICs). By focusing on clinically effective and practically implementable innovations in resource-limited settings, they ensure that progress in neurosurgery translates into broader access to care. Their study underscores the interconnectedness of our global community, highlighting that each individual's health is intrinsically linked to the health of all.

Unmet Need

The necessity for academic global neurosurgeons stems from the stark disparities in health outcomes observed worldwide, particularly in neurosurgical

Current Landscape

Quantifying the exact number of academic global neurosurgeons is challenging due to the dynamic nature of the field and the varying definitions of what constitutes an "academic global neurosurgeon."[4,5] However, it is clear that the current cadre, though expanding, needs to catch up to the global demand for specialized neurologic care, particularly in LMICs where the burden of neurosurgical conditions is disproportionately high.[12,30] The scarcity of trained professionals in these regions highlights a significant gap in the global health workforce, requiring urgent attention and strategic investment.[19,22] The growth of academic global neurosurgeons is crucial for addressing the immediate needs of underserved populations and building a sustainable framework for health equity that spans continents and cultures. Their presence and work are essential in academic institutions, hospitals, and research centers worldwide. Yet, the need far outstrips the supply, underscoring the urgency of expanding training and recruitment efforts in this field.

The impact of even a single academic global neurosurgeon cannot be overstated. Each new academic global neurosurgeon represents a step toward closing the gap in global neurosurgical care. Still, the path ahead requires a concerted effort from governments, educational institutions, health care organizations, and international bodies to scale up the training and deployment of these vital health care professionals. By increasing the number of academic global neurosurgeons, we enhance our collective ability to respond to the neurosurgical needs of populations worldwide, particularly in areas where access to care is limited. This expansion is not just about numbers; it is about building a global community of health care professionals dedicated to equity, collaboration, and innovation to achieve better health outcomes for all.

Imagine a world where academic global neurosurgeons are as common as the need for their services. Their focus would be as diverse as the challenges they confront, from conducting groundbreaking research in neurosurgical techniques that are affordable and accessible to training the next generation of surgeons in low-resource settings. They would advocate for policies prioritizing health equity and lead international collaborations that harness humanity's collective genius to solve our most pressing health crises.

DISCUSSION
Training Academic Global Neurosurgeons

Training the next generation of academic global neurosurgeons is a journey of transformation—a transformation of skill, perspective, and purpose. An academic global neurosurgeon must be skilled clinically and within global health, academia, and research. Training of neurosurgeons to be skilled surgically is not the focus here. Hence, the following outlines an approach to improving future academic global neurosurgeon skills in the above-mentioned areas.

Global health
Global health focuses on improving health equity, reducing disparities, and ensuring access to quality health care for all, regardless of geographic location, socioeconomic status, or other determinants.[31] Central to the field are the fundamental tenets of interdisciplinary collaboration, cultural humility, and a commitment to the principles of equity and justice. Global health endeavors to understand and address the complex interplay of factors contributing to health outcomes, including social, economic, environmental, and political determinants. It advocates for a comprehensive approach that goes beyond the treatment of diseases to include prevention, public health initiatives, and health system strengthening.[32]

An academic global neurosurgeon's journey starts here by learning and building upon the fundamental tenets of global health as an undergraduate, graduate student, medical student, and during their residency. Educational programs completed before or during medical school or integrated into their neurosurgery residency are critical. Degree-granting programs such as the Master of Public Health (MPH), Master of Science in Global Health (MScGH), and Master of Public Policy (MPP) are just a few examples of essential educational opportunities. These are not merely academic pursuits to add more letters to one's name or meant to serve as educational gatekeeping mechanisms but the foundation upon which our future leaders will build their understanding of the complexities of global health.[33]

The pursuit of the MPH, MScGH, and MPP degrees equips aspiring academic global neurosurgeons with a comprehensive understanding of the multifaceted nature of health challenges at a global scale. These programs delve into health's social, economic, and environmental determinants, providing students with the analytical tools and frameworks necessary to devise effective interventions. Through this education, they gain insights into the systemic barriers that impede access to care and learn strategies to overcome these obstacles. The curriculum fosters critical thinking, enabling students to evaluate health policies, programs, and practices through an equity lens.[34–36] This foundational knowledge is crucial for developing medically sound, culturally sensitive, and economically viable solutions, ensuring that health interventions are accessible to the most vulnerable populations.

Moreover, these programs offer future academic global neurosurgeons the opportunity to engage with a diverse cohort of peers and mentors, facilitating a rich exchange of ideas and experiences. This collaborative learning environment encourages sharing best practices and innovations in global health, thereby broadening students' perspectives and enriching their understanding of global health challenges. Fieldwork and research projects integrated into these programs allow students to apply theoretic knowledge to real-world contexts, further enhancing their skills in designing and implementing health interventions. These programs lay the groundwork for their future contributions to neurosurgery and global health, preparing them to make a tangible impact on communities worldwide.

Academics

The path continues with mastering the art of academia—grant writing, team leadership, and teaching. These skills are the tools with which our academic global neurosurgeons will carve out new frontiers in research, education, and collaboration. They will learn to navigate the intricacies of funding, inspire and guide diverse teams, and impart knowledge.

Securing funding through grant writing is a critical skill for academic global neurosurgeons, serving as the lifeblood that provides dedicated time outside of clinical responsibilities and supports research initiatives, educational programs, and outreach efforts.[37–39] Mastery in this area enables surgeons to translate visionary ideas into actionable projects, securing the resources necessary to explore innovative treatments, conduct impactful research, and implement programs that can change the trajectory of global neurosurgical care. The grant writing process involves articulating the significance and feasibility of proposed projects while understanding the priorities and guidelines of funding bodies. This skill ensures that academic global neurosurgeons can effectively communicate the value of their study, aligning their objectives with broader health goals and securing the support needed to advance their missions. Luckily, degree-granting programs and other educational opportunities have arisen within the global neurosurgery space to address this critical skill need.[40]

Leadership within academic and clinical settings is another cornerstone for academic global neurosurgeons, requiring a nuanced blend of inspiration, strategy, and empathy. Effective team leadership fosters collaboration and mutual respect among a multidisciplinary team of health care professionals, researchers, and educators. By cultivating a culture of inclusivity and innovation, academic global neurosurgeons can harness the collective expertise of their teams to overcome challenges and achieve common goals. Their leadership extends beyond the confines of their immediate surroundings, influencing the broader medical and global health communities through their commitment to mentorship, ethical practice, and advocacy for health equity.

Teaching is essential to the academic global neurosurgeon's role, embodying the commitment to passing knowledge and skills to the next generation of medical professionals. Through teaching, they not only disseminate the latest advancements in neurosurgery and global health but also instill a sense of responsibility and compassion among their students. This mentorship plays a pivotal role in shaping the future of the field, ensuring that upcoming surgeons are not only skilled clinicians but also thoughtful leaders who are prepared to address the complex health challenges of a globalized world.[41–44]

Moreover, integrating academics into the practice of global neurosurgery facilitates the continuous improvement of health care delivery through evidence-based practices and innovation. By engaging in research, academic global neurosurgeons contribute to the body of knowledge that informs best practices and policy development in neurosurgery and global health. Their study in academia supports the development of new surgical techniques, understanding of disease patterns, and strategies for effective health care delivery in diverse settings. This commitment to academics ensures that the field of global neurosurgery remains dynamic, responsive, and at the forefront of addressing the evolving health care needs of populations worldwide.

Research

At the heart of our endeavor lies research. From design to dissemination, our surgeons will become adept in the science of discovery. They will learn how to gather and analyze data and share their findings with the world, ensuring that their study transcends academic journals to tangible improvements in the lives of those they serve.

The foundation of impactful research in global neurosurgery is well-conceived research design. This involves formulating straightforward, relevant research questions and developing methodological approaches that are both rigorous and adaptable to the complexities of global health environments.[45–48] Academic global neurosurgeons must be versed in various research methodologies, from randomized controlled trials to qualitative studies, enabling them to address the multifaceted health challenges of different populations and settings. This skill set allows them to not only identify and address gaps in neurosurgical care but also test and refine interventions that are culturally and contextually appropriate. The research design process is iterative and collaborative, requiring continuous engagement with local communities, health care professionals, and stakeholders to ensure that research objectives are aligned with the needs and priorities of those they aim to serve.

Data collection through analysis forms the critical bridge between research questions and actionable insights. Academic global neurosurgeons must be adept at gathering high-quality data, employing quantitative and qualitative methods to capture the nuances of neurosurgical issues across diverse contexts. This involves navigating logistical challenges, ensuring ethical standards, and applying robust statistical and analytical techniques to interpret data accurately. Through rigorous data analysis, they contribute to a deeper understanding of disease epidemiology, intervention effectiveness, and health care delivery models, driving advancements in global neurosurgical care.

Dissemination of research findings is a crucial phase where knowledge is translated into practice and policy. Academic global neurosurgeons must excel in communicating their findings to various audiences, including the scientific community, policymakers, health care providers, and the public. This involves crafting compelling narratives highlighting their study's significance and implications for improving neurosurgical care and health outcomes. Through peer-reviewed publications, conferences, policy briefs, and community engagement, they ensure that their research does not remain siloed in academia but influences clinical practice, guides health policy, and raises stakeholder awareness. Effective dissemination amplifies the impact of their research, fostering a culture of knowledge sharing and collaboration that is essential for the progression of global neurosurgery.

Moreover, the research cycle in academic global neurosurgery is one of continuous learning and adaptation. By engaging in the full spectrum of research activities, from design to dissemination, academic global neurosurgeons contribute to the current body of knowledge and set the stage for future investigations. They inspire questions that push the boundaries of what is known, driving innovation and discovery in an ever-evolving field. Their commitment to research excellence paves the way for sustainable improvements in global neurosurgical care, ensuring that the most advanced and effective treatments are accessible to all, regardless of geographic or socioeconomic barriers.

Integration of Global Neurosurgery into Residency

Integrating global neurosurgery training into neurosurgery residencies worldwide requires a multifaceted approach, emphasizing the acquisition of surgical skills and a deep understanding of the global disparities in health care access and outcomes. This begins with developing curriculum components tailored to address global neurosurgery's unique challenges and needs. Such components should include modules on global health ethics, the social determinants of health, the principles of health equity, and the practicalities of delivering neurosurgical care in low-resource settings.[40] By embedding these topics into the residency curriculum, we cultivate a generation of neurosurgeons who are technically proficient, culturally humble, and committed to addressing health disparities.

Moreover, fostering partnerships between institutions in high-income countries and those in LMICs is essential for providing residents with firsthand experience in diverse clinical settings. These collaborations can facilitate exchange programs that allow residents to spend part of their training in settings that differ significantly from their primary learning environment. Such experiences are invaluable; they enhance surgical skills and adaptability and deepen residents' understanding of the global burden of neurosurgical diseases and the complexities of delivering care across different health systems.[49–51] These partnerships can also support capacity-building in underserved areas, creating a reciprocal relationship that benefits both the residents in training and the host communities.

The role of mentorship cannot be overstated in successfully integrating global neurosurgery into residencies. Mentorship by experienced global neurosurgeons provides residents with guidance, inspiration, and the opportunity to engage in global health research, advocacy, and clinical projects. These mentors can help navigate the complexities of planning and executing international collaborations, including securing funding, navigating ethical considerations, and ensuring sustainable impact. By establishing a mentorship framework, residency programs can create a supportive environment that encourages residents to pursue interests in global neurosurgery, fostering a culture of continuous learning and commitment to global health equity.

Lastly, leveraging technology and innovation presents a significant opportunity to enhance global neurosurgery training within residency programs. Telemedicine, virtual reality simulations, and online educational platforms can provide residents access to expert knowledge and technical training, transcending geographic limitations.[52–55] These technologies can facilitate virtual exchanges and collaborations, allowing residents to participate in case discussions, surgical planning, and educational seminars with peers and mentors worldwide. By integrating these innovative tools into residency training, we can expand the reach and impact of global neurosurgery education, preparing residents to become leaders in an increasingly interconnected field that relies on collaborative, multidisciplinary approaches to address the global challenges in neurosurgical care.

Creating Positions at Academic Institutions

Creating academic global neurosurgery positions within academic institutions worldwide necessitates a visionary approach that recognizes the dual imperative of clinical excellence and research innovation. The first step involves academic institutions acknowledging the value and necessity of integrating global health perspectives into their neurosurgery departments. This can be achieved by developing dedicated positions that explicitly combine clinical duties with research in global neurosurgery. These roles should be designed to allow surgeons to engage in meaningful clinical work, both within their home institutions and in partnerships with facilities in LMICs, while also dedicating significant time to research endeavors to address global neurosurgical challenges. By formalizing these positions, institutions signal their commitment to advancing global neurosurgery as a critical mission component.

To support the success of these positions, institutions must also commit to providing the necessary resources and infrastructure. This includes funding for research projects, access to global health training and mentorship programs, and logistical support for international collaboration. Financial models might consist of a mix of university funds, grants, and philanthropic contributions tailored to sustain the long-term viability of these positions. Equally important is creating an institutional culture that values global health equity, encouraging collaboration across departments and disciplines. This environment fosters interdisciplinary research, enhancing the depth and impact of studies to improve neurosurgical care in underserved regions. By investing in the necessary resources and fostering a supportive culture, academic institutions can empower global neurosurgeons to innovate and lead.

Furthermore, establishing robust partnerships with health care facilities and academic institutions in LMICs and even in low-resourced domestic settings is crucial. These partnerships should be based on mutual respect, equity, and shared goals, focusing on capacity building and sustainable development rather than one-sided assistance. For global neurosurgeons, such collaborations offer invaluable insights into the challenges and opportunities of providing neurosurgical care in diverse settings, enriching their research and clinical practice.[56] These partnerships also facilitate bilateral exchanges, allowing for the sharing of knowledge, skills, and resources. By prioritizing equitable partnerships, academic institutions can ensure that creating global neurosurgery positions leads to meaningful improvements in patient care and health systems strengthening worldwide.

Lastly, institutions must prioritize education and mentorship to nurture the next generation of academic global neurosurgeons. This includes incorporating global neurosurgery into the curriculum for medical students and residents and offering specialized fellowships and research opportunities in global neurosurgery. Mentoring programs that connect aspiring global neurosurgeons with experienced mentors can provide guidance, support, and inspiration. These educational initiatives should emphasize the importance of ethical engagement, cultural humility, and collaborative research, preparing trainees to navigate the complexities of global health work. By committing to the education and mentorship of future global neurosurgeons, academic institutions play a pivotal role in sustaining the growth and development of the field, ensuring a continuous pipeline of dedicated professionals ready to advance the mission of global neurosurgery.

SUMMARY

In an era marked by profound disparities in health care access and outcomes, the role of the academic global neurosurgeon emerges as a pivotal force for change, blending clinical excellence with a steadfast commitment to global health equity. These professionals stand at the vanguard of neurosurgery, extending their expertise beyond traditional boundaries to address the urgent needs of underserved populations worldwide. Their study is characterized by a multifaceted approach encompassing surgical care, education, research, and advocacy, ensuring that all share the benefits of medical advancements. Through a unique blend of clinical skills and a deep understanding of global health challenges, academic global neurosurgeons act as catalysts for change, working to bridge the gap between high-quality neurosurgical care and communities where such care is most needed.

A comprehensive training model integrating global health principles, research acumen, and leadership skills into neurosurgery residency programs is essential to cultivate the next generation of academic global neurosurgeons. This model emphasizes the importance of interdisciplinary learning, hands-on experience in diverse health care settings, and the development of strong partnerships between institutions across the globe.

By embedding global health education into the core of neurosurgical training, aspiring surgeons are equipped with the knowledge, skills, and perspectives necessary to navigate the complexities of global health challenges. Ultimately, this article underscores the imperative of creating academic positions and supportive infrastructures within institutions worldwide, fostering an environment where academic global neurosurgeons can thrive, innovate, and lead efforts to reduce health disparities, ensuring equitable neurosurgical care for all.

SUMMARY (CALL TO ACTION)

As we stand on the precipice of change, the vision of training the next generation of academic global neurosurgeons is not just an aspiration—it is an imperative. It is a commitment to the belief that where you live should not determine whether you live. Let us rise to this challenge in the spirit of unity, innovation, and compassion. Let us build a future where every individual has access to the neurosurgical care they need and deserve, no matter where they are born. Together, we can forge a new path, illuminated by the knowledge that in the pursuit of health, we are all connected, responsible, and beneficiaries of the boundless potential of academic global neurosurgery.

CLINICS CARE POINTS

Pearls

- Interdisciplinary collaboration is key: Successful academic global neurosurgeons thrive on interdisciplinary collaboration, which enhances their ability to address complex health challenges through diverse perspectives and expertise.
- Cultural humility enhances impact: Understanding and respecting cultural nuances improves the effectiveness of health care interventions.

- Research drives innovation: Engaging in rigorous research activities, especially those focused on prevalent health issues in low-resource settings, is crucial for academic global neurosurgeons.
- Education and mentorship are foundations for growth: Comprehensive training programs that include global health education, research methodologies, and leadership development are essential for preparing the next generation of academic global neurosurgeons. Mentorship, in particular, plays a pivotal role in guiding young surgeons through the complexities of global health engagement.
- Sustainable partnerships amplify impact: Establishing long-term, equitable partnerships with institutions and communities in LMICs is a cornerstone for successful global neurosurgery initiatives.

Pitfalls

- Underestimating local health systems: Ignoring the strengths and limitations of local health systems can lead to interventions that are not sustainable or effective in the long term.
- One-size-fits-all solutions: Applying solutions that worked in one setting to another without adapting to local contexts can lead to failure.
- Neglecting continuous education: Failing to stay updated with the latest global health research and neurosurgical techniques can limit an academic global neurosurgeon's ability to provide the best possible care and contribute to the field's advancement.
- Overlooking the importance of local partnerships: Working in isolation or without deep engagement with local partners can hinder the effectiveness and sustainability of health initiatives.
- Insufficient focus on health equity: Losing sight of the overarching goal of health equity can lead to initiatives that inadvertently perpetuate disparities.

DISCLOSURE

The authors have no relevant disclosures.

REFERENCES

1. Uche EO, Sundblom J, Uko UK, et al. Global neurosurgery over a 60-year period: Conceptual foundations, time reference, emerging Co-ordinates and prospects for collaborative interventions in low and middle income countries. Brain Spine 2022;2:101187.

2. Paradie E, Warman PI, Waguia-Kouam R, et al. The scope, growth, and inequities of the global neurosurgery literature: a bibliometric analysis. World Neurosurg 2022;167:e670–84.

3. Behmer Hansen RT, Behmer Hansen RA, Behmer VA, et al. Update on the global neurosurgery movement: A systematic review of international vernacular, research trends, and authorship. J Clin Neurosci 2020;79:183–90.

4. Andrews RJ. What's in a Name? "Global Neurosurgery" in the 21st Century. World Neurosurg 2020; 143:336–8.

5. Park KB, Johnson WD, Dempsey RJ. Global Neurosurgery: The Unmet Need. World Neurosurg 2016; 88:32–5.

6. Fuller AT, Arraez MA, Haglund MM. The role of nonprofit and academic institutions in global neurosurgery. In: Germano IM, editor. Neurosurgery and global health. Springer International Publishing; 2022. p. 309–24.

7. Gandy K, Castillo H, Rocque BG, et al. Neurosurgical training and global health education: systematic review of challenges and benefits of in-country programs in the care of neural tube defects. Neurosurg Focus 2020;48(3):E14.

8. Kanmounye US, Shlobin NA, Dempsey RJ, et al. Foundation for International Education in Neurosurgery: The Next Half-Century of Service Through Education. JGNS 2021;1(1):68–72. Available at: https://medcytjournals.com/index.php/JGNS/article/view/236. [Accessed 5 March 2024].

9. Ferraris KP, Matsumura H, Wardhana DPW, et al. The state of neurosurgical training and education in East Asia: analysis and strategy development for this frontier of the world. Neurosurg Focus 2020;48(3):E7.

10. Leidinger A, Extremera P, Kim EE, et al. The challenges and opportunities of global neurosurgery in East Africa: the Neurosurgery Education and Development model. Neurosurg Focus 2018;45(4):E8.

11. Fuller A, Tran T, Muhumuza M, et al. Building neurosurgical capacity in low and middle income countries. eNeurologicalSci 2015;3:1–6. Search Google Scholar Export Citation. Available at: https://scholar.google.ca/scholar?cluster=15294684988227476232&hl=en&as_sdt=0,5&sciodt=0,5.

12. Dewan MC, Rattani A, Gupta S, et al. Estimating the global incidence of traumatic brain injury. J Neurosurg 2018;1–18.

13. Quinsey C, Eaton J, Northam W, et al. Challenges and opportunities for effective data collection in global neurosurgery: traumatic brain injury surveillance experience in Malawi. Neurosurg Focus 2018;45(4):E10.

14. Kolias AG, Rubiano AM, Figaji A, et al. Traumatic brain injury: global collaboration for a global challenge. Lancet Neurol 2019;18(2):136–7.

15. Garcia RM, Ghotme KA, Arynchyna-Smith A, et al. Global Neurosurgery: Progress and Resolutions at the 75th World Health Assembly. Neurosurgery 2023;93(3):496–501.

16. Shlobin NA, Roach JT, Kancherla V, et al. The role of neurosurgeons in global public health: the case of folic acid fortification of staple foods to prevent spina bifida. J Neurosurg Pediatr 2023;31(1):8–15.

17. Veerappan VR, Gabriel PJ, Shlobin NA, et al. Global Neurosurgery in the Context of Global Public Health Practice–A Literature Review of Case Studies. World Neurosurg 2022;165:20–6.

18. Servadei F, Rossini Z, Nicolosi F, et al. The Role of Neurosurgery in Countries with Limited Facilities: Facts and Challenges. World Neurosurg 2018;112: 315–21.

19. Dewan MC, Rattani A, Fieggen G, et al. Global neurosurgery: the current capacity and deficit in the provision of essential neurosurgical care. Executive Summary of the Global Neurosurgery Initiative at the Program in Global Surgery and Social Change. J Neurosurg 2018;130(4):1055–64. Available at: https://thejns.org/view/journals/j-neurosurg/130/4/article-p1055.xml.

20. Mukhopadhyay S, Punchak M, Rattani A, et al. The global neurosurgical workforce: a mixed-methods assessment of density and growth. J Neurosurg 2019;1–7.

21. Ukachukwu AEK, Seas A, Petitt Z, et al. Assessing the Success and Sustainability of Global Neurosurgery Collaborations: Systematic Review and Adaptation of the Framework for Assessment of InteRNational Surgical Success Criteria. World Neurosurg 2022; 167:111–21.

22. Ukachukwu AEK, Still MEH, Seas A, et al. Fulfilling the specialist neurosurgical workforce needs in Africa: a systematic review and projection toward 2030. J Neurosurg 2023;138(4):1102–13.

23. Fuller A, Haglund M. The Importance of Collaboration in Global Neurosurgery. J Global Neurosurg 2021;1(1):78–9. Available at: http://198.12.226.205/index.php/jgn/article/view/238. [Accessed 1 October 2021].

24. Almeida JP, Velásquez C, Karekezi C, et al. Global neurosurgery: models for international surgical education and collaboration at one university. Neurosurg Focus 2018;45(4):E5.

25. Rehman AU, Ahmed A, Zaheer Z, et al. International neurosurgery: The role for collaboration. Int J Med Pharm Res 2023;4(1):15–24.

26. Cheyuo C, Hodaie M. Editorial. Neurosurgical capacity-building in Africa: how do we build an equitable future? J Neurosurg 2022;138(4):1098–9.

27. Rolle M, Ammar A, Park KB. Global Neurosurgery: A call to Action. JGNS 2021;1(1):86–8. Available at: https://medcytjournals.com/index.php/JGNS/article/view/243. [Accessed 5 March 2024].

28. Kanmounye US, Ghomsi N, Djiofack D, et al. The implications of global Neurosurgery for low- and middle-income countries: The case of Cameroon. J Neurosurg 2020;6:93–100.

29. Shlobin NA, Savage S, Savage A, et al. The World Neurosurgery Global Champions Program: First-Year Experience of a Model Initiative for Reducing Disparities in Global Neurosurgical Literature. World Neurosurg 2023. https://doi.org/10.1016/j.wneu.2023.06.015.

30. GBD 2016 Traumatic Brain Injury and Spinal Cord Injury Collaborators. Global, regional, and national burden of traumatic brain injury and spinal cord injury, 1990-2016: a systematic analysis for the Global Burden of Disease Study 2016. Lancet Neurol 2019;18(1):56–87.

31. Garay J, Harris L, Walsh J. Global health: evolution of the definition, use and misuse of the term. Face à face, 12 | 2013 La santé globale existe-t-elle ? Santé, science et politique aux Suds 2013;(12). Available at: http://journals.openedition.org/faceaface/745. [Accessed 5 March 2024].

32. Koplan JP, Bond TC, Merson MH, et al. Towards a common definition of global health. Lancet 2009; 373(9679):1993–5.

33. Shlobin NA, Kanmounye US, Ozair A, et al. Educating the Next Generation of Global Neurosurgeons: Competencies, Skills, and Resources for Medical Students Interested in Global Neurosurgery. World Neurosurg 2021;155:150–9.

34. Jacobsen KH, Zeraye HA, Bisesi MS, et al. Master of Public Health concentrations in global health in 2020: Preparing culturally competent professionals to address health disparities in the context of globalization. Health Promot Pract 2021;22(4):574–84.

35. Jacobsen KH, Li X, Gartin M, et al. Master of Science (MS) and master of Arts (MA) degrees in global health: Applying interdisciplinary research skills to the study of globalization-related health disparities. Pedagogy Health Promot 2020;6(1):14–22.

36. Leon JS, Winskell K, McFarland DA, et al. A case-based, problem-based learning approach to prepare master of public health candidates for the complexities of global health. Am J Publ Health 2015; 105(Suppl 1):S92–6.

37. Hauptman JS, Chow DS, Martin NA, et al. Research productivity in neurosurgery: trends in globalization, scientific focus, and funding. J Neurosurg 2011; 115(6):1262–72.

38. Griswold DP, Khan AA, Chao TE, et al. Neurosurgical Randomized Trials in Low- and Middle-Income Countries. Neurosurgery 2020;87(3):476–83.

39. Rolle ML, Garba DL, Kerry VB, et al. Commentary: the importance of increased funding opportunities to empower global neurosurgeons from low-middle income Countries. Neurosurgery 2021;89(4): E235–6.

40. Rolle ML, Zaki M, Parker T, et al. Global Neurosurgery Education in United States Residency Programs. World Neurosurg 2020;141:e815–9.

41. Minta KJ, Sescu D, Da Luz D, et al, GloMNMS Study Group Collaborators. Global Mentorship in Neurosurgery for Medical Students Study (the GloMNMS Study): a multinational multi-institutional cross-sectional audit. BMJ Open 2023;13(8):e071696.

42. Akhigbe T, Zolnourian A, Bulters D. Mentoring models in neurosurgical training: Review of literature. J Clin Neurosci 2017;45:40–3.

43. Koller GM, Reardon T, Kortz MW, et al. Shared objective mentorship via virtual research and education initiatives for medical students and residents in neurosurgery: A systematic review and methodological discussion of the Neurosurgery Education and Research Virtual Group experience. World Neurosurg 2023;172:20–33.

44. Hoffman C, Härtl R, Shlobin NA, et al. Future directions for global clinical neurosurgical training: challenges and opportunities. World Neurosurg 2022; 166:e404–18.

45. Whiffin CJ, Smith BG, Esene IN, et al. Neurosurgeons' experiences of conducting and disseminating clinical research in low-income and middle-income countries: a reflexive thematic analysis. BMJ Open 2021; 11(9):e051806.

46. Ham EI, Kim J, Kanmounye US, et al. Cohesion between research literature and health system level efforts to address global neurosurgical inequity: a scoping review. World Neurosurg 2020;143:e88–105.

47. Esene IN, Mbuagbaw L, Dechambenoit G, et al. Misclassification of case-control studies in neurosurgery and proposed solutions. World Neurosurg 2018;112:233–42.

48. Esene IN, Ngu J, El Zoghby M, et al. Case series and descriptive cohort studies in neurosurgery: the confusion and solution. Childs Nerv Syst 2014; 30(8):1321–32.

49. Starke RM, Asthagiri AR, Jane JA Sr, et al. Neurological surgery training abroad as a progression to the final year of training and transition to independent practice. J Grad Med Educ 2014;6(4):715–20.

50. Starke RM, Jane JA Jr, Asthagiri AR, et al. International rotations and resident education. J Neurosurg 2015;122(2):237–9.

51. Lundy P, Miller C, Woodrow S. Current US neurosurgical resident involvement, interest, and barriers in global neurosurgery. Neurosurg Focus 2020;48(3):E16.

52. Higginbotham G. Virtual connections: improving global neurosurgery through immersive technologies. Front Surg 2021;8:629963.

53. Safa A, De Biase G, Ramos-Fresnedo A, et al. Interactive neurosurgery lecture series: a global education platform of tele-teaching during the coronavirus disease 2019 pandemic and beyond. World Neurosurg 2022;166:e731–40.

54. Martini ML, Shrivastava RK, Kellner CP, et al. Evaluation of a role for virtual neurosurgical education for medical students over 2 years of a global pandemic. World Neurosurg 2022;166:e253–62.

55. El-Ghandour NMF, Ezzat AAM, Zaazoue MA, et al. Virtual learning during the COVID-19 pandemic: a turning point in neurosurgical education. Neurosurg Focus 2020;49(6):E18.

56. Lartigue JW, Dada OE, Haq M, et al. Emphasizing the role of neurosurgery within global health and national health systems: a call to action. Front Surg 2021;8:690735.

UNITED STATES POSTAL SERVICE®

Statement of Ownership, Management, and Circulation
(All Periodicals Publications Except Requester Publications)

1. Publication Title
NEUROSURGERY CLINICS OF NORTH AMERICA

2. Publication Number
010 – 548

3. Filing Date
9/18/2024

4. Issue Frequency
JAN, APR, JUL, OCT

5. Number of Issues Published Annually
4

6. Annual Subscription Price
$465.00

7. Complete Mailing Address of Known Office of Publication (Not printer) (Street, city, county, state, and ZIP+4®)
ELSEVIER INC.
230 Park Avenue, Suite 800
New York, NY 10169

Contact Person
Malathi Samayan

Telephone (Include area code)
91-44-4299-4507

8. Complete Mailing Address of Headquarters or General Business Office of Publisher (Not printer)
ELSEVIER INC.
230 Park Avenue, Suite 800
New York, NY 10169

9. Full Names and Complete Mailing Addresses of Publisher, Editor, and Managing Editor (Do not leave blank)

Publisher (Name and complete mailing address)
Dolores Meloni, ELSEVIER INC.
1600 JOHN F KENNEDY BLVD. SUITE 1600
PHILADELPHIA, PA 19103-2899

Editor (Name and complete mailing address)
STACY EASTMAN, ELSEVIER INC.
1600 JOHN F KENNEDY BLVD. SUITE 1600
PHILADELPHIA, PA 19103-2899

Managing Editor (Name and complete mailing address)
PATRICK MANLEY, ELSEVIER INC.
1600 JOHN F KENNEDY BLVD. SUITE 1600
PHILADELPHIA, PA 19103-2899

10. Owner (Do not leave blank. If the publication is owned by a corporation, give the name and address of the corporation immediately followed by the names and addresses of all stockholders owning or holding 1 percent or more of the total amount of stock. If not owned by a corporation, give the names and addresses of the individual owners. If owned by a partnership or other unincorporated firm, give its name and address as well as those of each individual owner. If the publication is published by a nonprofit organization, give its name and address.)

Full Name	Complete Mailing Address
WHOLLY OWNED SUBSIDIARY OF REED/ELSEVIER, US HOLDINGS	1600 JOHN F KENNEDY BLVD. SUITE 1600 PHILADELPHIA, PA 19103-2899

11. Known Bondholders, Mortgagees, and Other Security Holders Owning or Holding 1 Percent or More of Total Amount of Bonds, Mortgages, or Other Securities. If none, check box. ▶ ☐ None

Full Name	Complete Mailing Address
N/A	

12. Tax Status (For completion by nonprofit organizations authorized to mail at nonprofit rates) (Check one)
The purpose, function, and nonprofit status of this organization and the exempt status for federal income tax purposes:
☒ Has Not Changed During Preceding 12 Months
☐ Has Changed During Preceding 12 Months (Publisher must submit explanation of change with this statement)

PS Form 3526, July 2014 [Page 1 of 4 (see instructions page 4)] PSN: 7530-01-000-9931   PRIVACY NOTICE: See our privacy policy on www.usps.com.

---

13. Publication Title
NEUROSURGERY CLINICS OF NORTH AMERICA

14. Issue Date for Circulation Data Below
JULY 2024

15. Extent and Nature of Circulation

		Average No. Copies Each Issue During Preceding 12 Months	No. Copies of Single Issue Published Nearest to Filing Date
a. Total Number of Copies (Net press run)		112	104
b. Paid Circulation (By Mail and Outside the Mail)	(1) Mailed Outside-County Paid Subscriptions Stated on PS Form 3541 (Include paid distribution above nominal rate, advertiser's proof copies, and exchange copies)	71	72
	(2) Mailed In-County Paid Subscriptions Stated on PS Form 3541 (Include paid distribution above nominal rate, advertiser's proof copies, and exchange copies)	0	0
	(3) Paid Distribution Outside the Mails Including Sales Through Dealers and Carriers, Street Vendors, Counter Sales, and Other Paid Distribution Outside USPS®	25	21
	(4) Paid Distribution by Other Classes of Mail Through the USPS (e.g., First-Class Mail®)	10	5
c. Total Paid Distribution (Sum of 15b (1), (2), (3), and (4)) ▶		106	98
d. Free or Nominal Rate Distribution (By Mail and Outside the Mail)	(1) Free or Nominal Rate Outside-County Copies included on PS Form 3541	5	5
	(2) Free or Nominal Rate In-County Copies Included on PS Form 3541	0	0
	(3) Free or Nominal Rate Copies Mailed at Other Classes Through the USPS (e.g., First-Class Mail)	0	0
	(4) Free or Nominal Rate Distribution Outside the Mail (Carriers or other means)	1	1
e. Total Free or Nominal Rate Distribution (Sum of 15d (1), (2), (3) and (4)) ▶		6	6
f. Total Distribution (Sum of 15c and 15e) ▶		112	104
g. Copies not Distributed (See Instructions to Publishers #4 (page #3)) ▶		0	0
h. Total (Sum of 15f and g) ▶		112	104
i. Percent Paid (15c divided by 15f times 100) ▶		94.63%	94.23%

* If you are claiming electronic copies, go to line 16 on page 3. If you are not claiming electronic copies, skip to line 17 on page 3.

PS Form 3526, July 2014 (Page 2 of 4)

16. Electronic Copy Circulation

		Average No. Copies Each Issue During Preceding 12 Months	No. Copies of Single Issue Published Nearest to Filing Date
a. Paid Electronic Copies	▶		
b. Total Paid Print Copies (Line 15c) + Paid Electronic Copies (Line 16a)	▶		
c. Total Print Distribution (Line 15f) + Paid Electronic Copies (Line 16a)	▶		
d. Percent Paid (Both Print & Electronic Copies) (16b divided by 16c × 100)	▶		

☒ I certify that 50% of all my distributed copies (electronic and print) are paid above a nominal price.

17. Publication of Statement of Ownership
☒ If the publication is a general publication, publication of this statement is required. Will be printed in the OCTOBER 2024 issue of this publication.   ☐ Publication not required.

18. Signature and Title of Editor, Publisher, Business Manager, or Owner

Malathi Samayan   Date 9/18/2024

Malathi Samayan - Distribution Controller

I certify that all information furnished on this form is true and complete. I understand that anyone who furnishes false or misleading information on this form or who omits material or information requested on the form may be subject to criminal sanctions (including fines and imprisonment) and/or civil sanctions (including civil penalties).

PS Form 3526, July 2014 (Page 3 of 4)   PRIVACY NOTICE: See our privacy policy on www.usps.com

Moving?

Make sure your subscription moves with you!

To notify us of your new address, find your **Clinics Account Number** (located on your mailing label above your name), and contact customer service at:

Email: journalscustomerservice-usa@elsevier.com

800-654-2452 (subscribers in the U.S. & Canada)
314-447-8871 (subscribers outside of the U.S. & Canada)

Fax number: 314-447-8029

Elsevier Health Sciences Division
Subscription Customer Service
3251 Riverport Lane
Maryland Heights, MO 63043

*To ensure uninterrupted delivery of your subscription, please notify us at least 4 weeks in advance of move.

Printed and bound by CPI Group (UK) Ltd, Croydon, CR0 4YY

08/05/2025

01864724-0017